"This delightful book is an integration of the author's experience both as classroom teacher and a yoga teacher. Clearly and succinctly, Cohen Harper shows how dynamic mindfulness skills such as yoga, breathing techniques, and meditation can help children flourish in school and in life. It is as much a guide for children as it is for the adults around them, helping all with stress management, self-awareness, and emotion regulation. With one in two children dropping out of our inner-city schools, there is no time like the present for widespread dissemination and adoption of these foundational, time-tested, transformative practices."

—**Bidyut K. Bose, PhD**, founder and executive director of the Niroga Institute at www.niroga.org

"Bridging the science of yoga for children with practical application, Cohen Harper demonstrates her extensive experience as an educator and kids' yoga teacher with this indispensable resource for parents, educators, therapists, and other adults who care deeply for the children in their lives. Whether you are new to the practice or an experienced Yogi, Little Flower's five essential elements of yoga for children will provide you with an accessible framework for sharing yoga with kids. This thoughtfully written book includes information such as how to set up a yoga space and which props to use; dozens of child-friendly meditation activities, breathing exercises, and poses; and the science behind it all, providing the reader with a comprehensive approach to promoting mindfulness, focus, and resilience."

—**Lisa Flynn**, founder of ChildLight Yoga and Yoga 4 Classrooms and author of the *Yoga 4 Classrooms Card Deck* and *Yoga for Children*

"The curriculum's fluid and organic incorporation of 'connect, breathe, move, focus, and relax' ensure that students will have a full and joyful experience each time they are on the mat and practicing yoga. My favorite parts are the laughter, the connection, and the 'a-ha' moments that are a part of her classes every day!"

—**Susan Verde**, parent

"*Little Flower Yoga for Kids* is an excellent guidebook for parents and educators seeking a program that will help children with focus and balance. Cohen Harper does a masterful job of simplifying the practices of yoga while maintaining the integrity of the tradition. She divides activities into handy categories like connecting, breathing, moving, focusing, and relaxing—all of which offer a comprehensive set of tools for parents to support the growth of the whole family. The perfect manual for making kids and parents more aware of the magic of mindfulness."

> —**Beryl Bender Birch**, director and founder of the Hard and the Soft Yoga Institute and the Give Back Yoga Foundation

"*Little Flower Yoga for Kids* is a wonderful introduction to present-moment awareness and mindfulness through a grounded and playful yoga practice. It is an inspiring resource for children and their parents."

> —**Sharon Salzberg**, author of *Real Happiness* and *Lovingkindness*

"I recommend this book to anyone interested in learning practical ways to integrate health and wellness into the lives of children. Even someone with no prior experience in yoga or mindfulness can utilize this content immediately to bring more balance to daily home life. Cohen Harper masterfully weaves theory and practice in a format that dispels any mystery around these ancient practices, making them accessible for folks wanting to find a little more focus and peace."

> —**Abby Wills, MA**, cofounder of Shanti Generation

"This book is infused with joy! Every page offers wisdom and essential skills with a delightful, gentle playfulness. Jennifer Cohen Harper shares the historical foundations of yoga and mindfulness and the complex neuroscience regarding their benefits in simple, accessible writing. The joyful process of sharing these sweet practices with your child will have profound benefits for both your child and you."

> —**Amy Saltzman, MD**

"This resource will empower school staff and students, and makes a solid contribution to the school yoga-mindfulness movement."

> —**Karma Carpenter Shea**, founder of the International Association for School Yoga and Mindfulness at k-12yoga.org

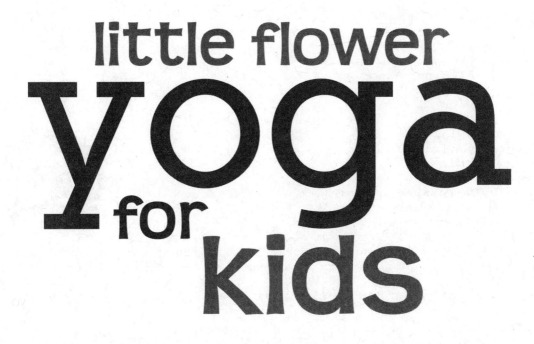

little flower yoga for kids

A Yoga and Mindfulness Program to Help Your Child Improve Attention and Emotional Balance

Jennifer Cohen Harper, MA, E-RCYT

New Harbinger Publications, Inc.

Publisher's Note

Distributed in Canada by Raincoast Books

Copyright © 2013 by Jennifer Cohen Harper
        New Harbinger Publications, Inc.
        5674 Shattuck Avenue
        Oakland, CA 94609
        www.newharbinger.com

Cover design by Amy Shoup
Interior design by Michele Waters-Kermes
Acquired by Tesilya Hanauer
Edited by Marisa Solís
Illustrations by Julie Olson, www.julieolsonillustrator.com
Cover & author photos: Lynda Shenkman Curtis

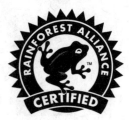

The full text for "Guiding Principles for Sharing Yoga with Your Child" was previously published on elephantjournal.com and is reprinted with permission from *Elephant Journal,* http://elephantjournal.com.

The full text for "Practice Yoga, Parent Better" and "A Guide to Compassionate Parenting" is excerpted from a letter by Kate Gilbane and printed with her permission.

Library of Congress Cataloging-in-Publication Data on file

Printed in the United States of America

15   14   13

10   9   8   7   6   5   4   3   2   1

First printing

For Isabelle

My happiest of happies. My newest teacher.

Contents

Acknowledgments vii

Foreword ix

Introduction 1

1   Understand 7

2   Explore 17

3   Get Started 29

4   Connect 39
     Layers of Sound 43
     Walking Meditation 45
     Mindful Eating 47
     Checking In 50
     Emotion Jar 55
     Caring Feelings 57
     I Am In Charge Mantra 59

5   Breathe 63
     Balloon Breath 68
     Heart and Belly Breath 71
     Langhana and Brahmana Breath 73
     Alternate-Nostril Breathing 76
     Back-to-Back Breathing 79

6   Move 83
     Warming Up: Cat, Cow, and Twist Poses 86
     A Place to Rest: Child's Pose 89
     Grounding: Mountain Pose 90
     Grounding: Malasana 92

Grounding: Seated Forward Bends 94

Strength: Warrior Poses 98

Strength: Moving Lunges 104

Strength: Boat Pose 108

Balance: Tree Pose 110

Balance: Side Plank Pose 112

Balance: Flower Pose 114

Balance: Half Moon Pose 116

Final Relaxation: Savasana 118

7   Focus 121

Exploring Your Drishti 124

Expanding-Energy Meditation 126

Single-Pointed Focus 128

Thought River Meditation 130

8   Relax 133

Legs Up the Wall Pose 136

Supported Reclined Bound-Ankle Pose 138

Guided Visualization 140

Tense and Let Go: Yoga Nidra 142

9   Putting It All Together 145

From Sitting to Standing: No-Hands Stand 150

From Standing to Sitting: Tiptoe Pose to Squatting 151

From Sitting to Reclining: Smallest You to Biggest You 152

Bringing Energy Up (Gently): Waking Up Your Body 154

Bringing Energy Down: Rag Doll Pose 155

Coming Back to Neutral: Simple Twist 156

10   Support for Parents 159

Appendix: Talking with Teachers 169

Recommended Reading 173

References 177

Acknowledgments

This book was written during a wonderfully joyful and exciting—and also quite challenging—time in my life: my pregnancy and the first six months of my daughter's life. It would not have been possible without a tremendous amount of support, encouragement, and love.

Thank you to the team at New Harbinger: Wendy Millstine, for seeking me out and planting the seeds of this collaboration; Tesilya Hanauer for your guidance, support, and advocacy; Angela Autry Gorden, for your help during Tesilya's own early months with her baby; Jess Beebe and Nicola Skidmore for your insightful and extremely useful feedback; the entire marketing team—particularly Julienne Bennett, Rachel Rogers, Karen Hathaway, Bevin Donahue, and Adia Colar—for your dedication to getting this book to its audience; Heather Garnos, Susan Alexander, Julie Olson, Heather Garnos, Michele Waters, and Amy Shoup for making sure the book looks its best; and Marisa Solís, for your graceful and thorough editing—it made the book better.

Kelly McGonigal and Gina Biegel were early supporters of this book when it was just in the proposal stage, and I'm grateful for both of their valuable advice. Tremendous thanks also to Dan Siegel for his time and support. Huge amounts of gratitude and love to all of the Little Flower Yoga teachers, particularly Kate Reil. You have been instrumental in shaping the course of our programming, and your knowledge, experience, skills, and feedback have continued to help me learn and grow. Thank you, Kelly Britton—your early words of simple encouragement made a big impact and set me firmly on this path.

Huge thanks to Mayuri Gonzalez, photographer Lynda Shenkman Curtis, and the kids of Prasanthi Studio for their work on the cover. Naiya Gonzalez, Pierce Gayle, Isabella Garcia, Alyssa Domenici, Leo Garcia, Annabelle Mount, Benjamin Malejko, and Mason Sznip—amazing yogis and superstar models!

Kate Gilbane, Susan Verde, and Tara Vanselow: Thank you for your valuable feedback as moms and yoga teachers, and your thoughts on working with your children's teachers. Kate, your contributions to the book are amazing. Thank you for your honesty and eloquence.

My family has proven time and time again to be a never-ending well of love, support, and help! Thank you to George for your advice and thoughtfulness; Jodie for your non-stop love and flying three thousand miles to babysit(!); and to Laureli, Ally, and Zach, for your encouragement and opinions (Laureli and Ally you are the best sisters ever!). Mom and Dad, you guys are the best. Thank you for a lifetime of feeling loved, respected, supported, and inspired. There is no way that Little Flower Yoga or this book could have happened without you, and I am grateful all the time. To my husband, Larry, for love, patience, help, advice, clean laundry, and being the most amazing partner possible, thank you one thousand thank-yous.

And of course, I am constantly grateful for the kids that have come into my life and taught me so much during the past ten years. Every time I feel like I've got a handle on this work, I seem to meet a child who challenges me to learn something new, think more creatively, open my heart a little wider, and become a better version of myself.

Foreword

It is a pleasure to say a few words to invite you into the wonderful world of Jennifer Harper Cohen's *Little Flower Yoga for Kids*. Our gentle and experienced author guides us on a journey into the artful practice and practical science of yoga for children. But this gem of a book is more than simply a useful set of carefully-described "how-to" instructions to get even a novice like me to try out the positions and moves. It is a step-by-step map to help you, as a parent or teacher, make this body-centered mindfulness practice a regular part of your life with the kids you care for.

For thousands of years, wisdom traditions have taught us that paying attention to the present moment has powerful positive effects on our health. In this new millennium, science has found empirically-validated support for these ancient claims that what we do with our minds and our bodies influences our well-being and our happiness. There are many ways to learn to pay attention to our moment-by-moment experience with openness and kind regard. Mindfulness comes in many forms. For children, the time-tested practices of yoga are a wonderful gateway into this world of mindful awareness.

With the digital distractions of modern times pulling our attention to visual and auditory stimuli of all sorts and all speeds, we've never before had such an urgent need for accessible methods to take "time-in" to focus the mind's attention on the inner world. This sea inside includes both the sensations in our bodies and the feelings and thoughts of our minds. When we focus inward and take time to cultivate our inner vision—what I call "mindsight"—we develop specific circuits in our brains that support our abilities to balance our emotions, focus our attention, pause before acting on impulses, and increase our compassion for others and ourselves.

Participating in the stretches and positions of yoga is far more than just a body workout. (But it does work the body, so if you have any concerns about your child's medical limitations, please check with your health care provider first.) When we help our kids learn the foundations of yoga, we are inviting them not only to position and move the body in certain ways but to focus attention on the sensations of the body. This does at least two things. One is that it makes it essential to focus inward and develop a strengthened sense of attention. That's a great thing just by itself. But a second skill is that we are helping kids develop is something called "interoception"—the perception of the interior of the body. The specific circuitry of interoception involves a central set of connections in the brain that support both self-awareness and empathy. The more interoceptive skills we develop, the better we know our selves and understand and connect with others.

You may find that hard to believe—that focusing attention on the present moment's sensations of the body in a mindfulness practice like yoga can actually change the circuits in the brain. But now, we not only know that this is true; we also know that being present for what is happening right now—focusing attention on life as it unfolds and not being distracted by multiple layers of external stimuli—actually supports our health in a number of ways. Studies of various mindfulness trainings reveal that our immune function is better when we learn to be present; and mindfulness even elevates an enzyme that maintains the integrity of our chromosomes.

And, if I am really being present here, I have to say that we have gotten much more out of mindfulness than just those two benefits. Remarkably, being present like this has also been shown to help us concentrate, balance emotion, and be more resilient in the face of challenges. And it has also been shown to make us happier. No kidding.

So why not offer this to your children? If mine were young, I'd get down on the floor with them and start. The truth is, now my older, out-of-the-house adolescents take me to yoga classes up at their school. Live and learn!

Enjoy the pages ahead, and breathe in these precious moments with your children. The days may sometimes feel so long, but believe me, their years at home are short. Savor them and enjoy!

—Daniel J. Siegel, MD
Author of *Mindsight, The Developing Mind, The Whole-Brain Child, Parenting from the Inside Out* and *Brainstorm*
Executive Director, Mindsight Institute
Clinical Professor, UCLA School of Medicine

Introduction

Thank you for your interest in sharing yoga and mindfulness with the children in your life. By reading this book you are starting on a journey that has the potential to improve the day-to-day well-being of your child and your family as a whole. You may have picked up this book because a child you care about is struggling. He may be having a hard time focusing, regulating his emotions, or communicating his feelings. He may have even been diagnosed with attention deficit/hyperactivity disorder (ADHD) or another condition that makes daily life more challenging.

This book is not about a problem or a disorder, however. This book is about strengthening your child's capacity for present-moment awareness and self-regulation. It's about increasing his connection with himself and the people around him, and ultimately about giving him a fuller and more enjoyable experience of life. All children—and most adults!—at times have difficulty focusing, being patient, and managing their emotions. This is perfectly normal but can also be very frustrating. Through the understanding and practice of yoga, your child—and you—will gain valuable life skills that can be used in school, at home, and in social situations.

The perspective of this book is that your child is a perfectly whole and healthy person, not that he is somehow in need of fixing. All of us have aspects of life that are challenging, and we all struggle to be the best versions of ourselves. Some of those challenges have names and some don't. Whether your child has been diagnosed with a disorder is less important than if he has a supportive community of adults who are paying attention in a compassionate way to his needs and strengths.

We can all get better at paying attention, and every child can benefit from these practices. This book is for parents who want to explore ways to give their children a full, healthy, and vibrant life. It offers a strength-based approach that embraces all children's capacity for greatness.

What Does It Mean to Pay Attention?

We often ask our children to pay attention. *Pay attention to your school work, pay attention to your father, pay attention to your teacher.* But we don't always have a clear idea of what we are actually asking of them. What does it mean to pay attention? Merriam-Webster's dictionary defines "attention" as "the act or state of applying the mind to something" (Merriam Webster, 11th ed., s.v. "attention").

William James (1950, 403), in *Principles of Psychology*, stated that "everyone knows what attention is. It is the taking possession by the mind, in clear and vivid form, of one out of what seem several simultaneously possible objects or trains of thought. . . . It implies withdrawal from some things in order to deal effectively with others, and is a condition which has a real opposite in the confused, dazed, scatterbrained state which in French is called distraction."

The fundamental challenge of paying attention is that there is so much to pay attention to! Our minds are constantly reacting to everything around us—taking it in and trying to make sense of it. Connecting to the past and projecting into the future. The human inclination is to process everything around us all the time in order to detect any possible threat or danger.

When we ask our children to pay attention to their homework or pay attention to what we are saying, what we really mean is something along the lines of *Stop thinking about all the other things that are important to you right now, no matter how you are feeling about those things—even if they are scary or confusing or are trying really hard to distract you. Focus exclusively on what I want you to focus on. Then respond in a way that is productive and socially appropriate.*

What we are asking our kids is very hard. For many children (and adults) it can seem impossible. In order to pay attention to any one thing, a person must be capable of filtering an enormous amount of other things: all of the external stimuli, and all of the internal thoughts, feelings, memories, and plans. We are always paying attention to something. What we are trying to do—and teach our kids how to do—is choose what we pay attention to and for how long we pay attention to it.

Why Yoga and Mindfulness?

Yoga and mindfulness are interrelated traditions that focus on the holistic wellness of the entire person. While many of us in the United States think of yoga as postures and breathing techniques, the full practice of yoga provides us with an accessible method of bringing the whole human—body, breath, and mind—into a balanced and healthy state. These practices work to systematically bring a greater amount of present-moment awareness to all areas of life.

There are some people who think that they practice mindfulness but not yoga, and some who think that they practice yoga but not mindfulness. In the fullest expression of both of these traditions, that is impossible. In chapter 2 we will spend more time discussing what yoga and mindfulness are, how they relate to each other, and what current research tells us about them. For now, know that mindfulness is the beginning and end of the yoga practice, and yoga is a particularly effective system for teaching yourself mindfulness—what Jon Kabat-Zinn (1994) describes as a nonjudgmental present-moment awareness and the capacity to act based on that awareness.

Many of our children are living a life dictated by their impulses. Yoga provides us with a set of tools for creating space between the input of life experiences and the output of our reactions. In that space, we can pay attention. We can notice what we are feeling, think for a moment, and make decisions. Once we can learn to find that space, we can use it to take control of our own lives.

There are many different types of yoga and many ways of practicing. In this book we are going to use a method of practice developed by Little Flower Yoga, a program that brings yoga and mindfulness into schools in New York. I founded LFY in 2006, in an effort to make these practices available and accessible to children regardless of circumstance or home life. The program reaches about one thousand children per week, challenging students to learn in new ways, make connections, and recognize their tremendous capacity to achieve. Before starting LFY, I worked for Harlem Children's Zone as both a kindergarten teacher and a yoga instructor, and I've been a student of Jivamukti yoga for more than twelve years.

My background in education informed the creation of the LFY program, and bringing the tools of yoga and mindfulness into schools is an amazing thing. But there is nothing that will impact a child more than what happens in his home on a daily basis. By taking the time to practice yoga and mindfulness with your child, you are giving him a strong foundation for lifelong wellness. This Little Flower Yoga teaching method is based on five elements that, in combination, create a complete experience of yoga and mindfulness in a way that can be tailored for the developmental needs of every child. Each one of these elements provides a crucial learning tool for helping children maintain their attention and develop the capacity for self-regulation.

Connect: Connect activities help children tune in and make sense of their experiences. They are practices that are used to develop mindful awareness of both the external world and the internal emotional state.

Breathe: The breath is one of the most powerful tools for self-regulation. Breathing activities help children learn to reduce anxiety, stabilize energy, and create a sense of safety and peace in the body.

Move: Move activities are based on yoga postures that help children maintain a state of alert engagement, where hyperactive behavior is minimized but the child still feels strong and energetic.

Focus: The Focus activities in this program provide deliberate exercises that teach children how to apply their focus in a step-by-step way, allowing for progressive improvement and experiences of success.

Relax: The final element of our program, Relax gives children tools for rest, relaxation, and restoration. Exhaustion is common in children, and we know that being tired makes everything else, including paying attention, much harder. These activities teach ways to rejuvenate even when you aren't sleeping.

Navigating this Book

This is a book that is meant to be absorbed in small pieces. It is a practical, tool-based approach to helping your child meet the challenges of the modern world while recognizing, supporting, and celebrating your child as an individual. The practices described in this book can be integrated into the life of your family over time, at a pace that feels enjoyable and sustainable.

The first chapter of this book takes a closer look at the science of focus, emotional regulation, and self-control. Chapter 2 will give you more information about yoga and mindfulness: what they are, how they relate to each other, and why they can help improve focus and emotional regulation. Chapter 3, Get Started, is a full guide for implementing this program with your child. It will give you all of the logistical information you need to work with your child safely and effectively.

The majority of this book is dedicated to practical activities within each of the five elements we've discussed. Chapters 4 through 8 will give you step-by-step instructions for introducing your child to these activities, along with ideas for integrating them into your child's daily life. Chapter 9, Putting It All Together, will give you suggestions for combining activities into full yoga sessions. Chapter 10 offers some thoughts on supporting your own wellness and dealing compassionately with the many challenges that parenting presents.

As you begin using yoga and mindfulness to change your child's experience of life, remember that these practices benefit everyone. The best way to make this experience enjoyable and meaningful for your child is to allow the practices described in this book to become a part of the lives of everyone in your family. The power of the activities is that, over time, they change the way you experience the world. By sharing these practices with your child, you will be able to better support her development and understand the experience she is having. As you read through this book, take the time to practice the activities yourself. Embrace them with an open mind and a spirit of curiosity and exploration—and your child is likely to do the same.

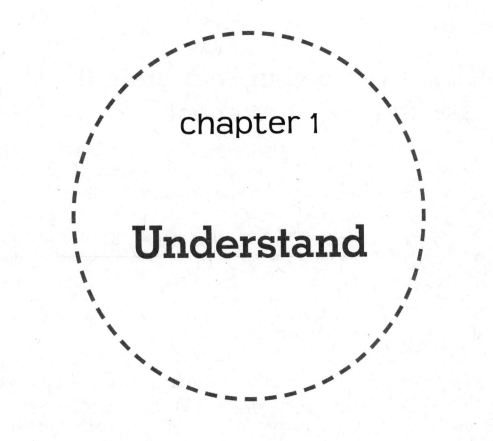

chapter 1

Understand

hoosing one thing to focus on, and maintaining that focus, sounds like a straightforward task, but it is enormously challenging when you consider all that has to happen in the brain and the body for it to take place. The human brain is amazing, with tremendous capacity and potential. Our brains work collaboratively with our entire bodies—our nervous system, our muscles, our organs—and coordinate a finely tuned balancing act among our thoughts, emotions, actions, reflexes, and habits in an effort to keep us alive and well. Understanding a bit about what is happening in your child's body and brain will help you understand more about what he needs in order to focus and pay attention more effectively.

What Has to Happen in Your Brain in Order For You to Pay Attention?

Your brain has many different parts, all of which have their own responsibilities. This differentiation means that in addition to communicating with the rest of your body, your brain has a tremendous amount of internal communication to do. How your brain handles this internal communication, and how the different parts of your brain learn to collaborate and coordinate with one another, is something that develops differently in every individual based on his or her life experiences. Your child's brain is absolutely unique (and so is yours).

The Protective Brain

The first part of the brain that we need to understand is also the part that develops first in our children. Sometimes called the *limbic area*, this is the lower part of the brain that is responsible for our emotions, reflexes, instincts, and basic bodily functions. This lower (sometimes called *primitive*) part of the brain is almost completely developed even before we are born. It is where our strongest emotions—such as fear, anger, love, and jealousy—live, and it is the most dominant part of the brain in children. Anytime we act based on an emotion or impulse, without giving much thought to either the logic of our action or its consequences, we are acting on the directions of this part of our brains. I find it helpful to think of the limbic area as the "Protective Brain," because it is always looking out for our safety and our immediate happiness. Sometimes it even tries to protect us from our own feelings and experiences if they get to be overwhelming.

One part of the limbic area that is particularly interesting to our conversation is the *amygdala*. The amygdala is a small part of the brain with a very big job. It is most responsible for protecting us in an emergency. It is what takes over when we feel like we are in danger and allows us to act immediately to protect ourselves, sometimes before the rest of our brain even knows what is happening. When we touch something hot and recoil from it instantly, it is the amygdala that is protecting us. When something makes us afraid, the amygdala tells our body to be on high alert, and it activates our sympathetic nervous system (the fight-flight-or-freeze response). Most of the time the amygdala is very useful, but sometimes in both children and adults it takes over even when there isn't a real emergency. This can happen for a lot of different reasons, which we'll discuss soon, but the effect can be that our actions don't reflect either the situation at hand or the best version of ourselves. When your child's amygdala takes control, some of your most frustrating parenting moments are likely to follow as tantrums, tears, and irrational behavior surge, while reason, negotiation, and compromise seem completely ineffective.

Although the Protective Brain is always on our side, standing up for our feelings and protecting us from danger, it doesn't always see the big picture. Then it becomes the "Overprotective Brain," keeping us from acting as our more thoughtful, compassionate, creative, and capable selves.

The Thoughtful Brain

In stark contrast to our Protective Brain is the *prefrontal cortex*, or what I call the "Thoughtful Brain." While the Protective Brain is emotion driven, the prefrontal cortex is busy thinking, planning, and imagining. In their 2011 book, *The Whole-Brain Child*, Dr. Daniel Siegel and Tina Payne Bryson refer to the prefrontal cortex as the "upstairs" brain, and note that when it is working well, a child can "regulate her emotions, consider consequences, think before acting, and consider how others feel" (Siegel and Bryson 2011, 40).

The prefrontal cortex is the part of our brain that can see the big picture. When our emotions and experiences are viewed through the lens of the prefrontal cortex, we can react to them with more thoughtful and rational behavior. The prefrontal cortex helps us take a long-term view of the world and consider more than just our immediate physical

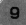

and emotional needs and desires. It works to help us control our impulses and consider the needs of others, helps motivate us when we are tired or frustrated or bored, and creatively works to solve problems.

There is a small part of the prefrontal cortex, called the *right orbitofrontal cortex*, that plays a big role in our discussion of increasing focus and attention. "From all the information about the external environment and internal body states entering our brain, the [orbitofrontal cortex] helps to pick out what to focus on" (Maté 2000, 78). It's interesting that this is also the part of our brain that hits the pause button on our emotional reactions to life experiences, delaying them long enough to "allow mature, more sophisticated responses to emerge" (Maté 2000, 79).

When it's functioning well, you can think of the orbitofrontal cortex as a sort of monitor over the amygdala, gathering information from the environment, from our bodies, and even from other parts of the brain, and deciding whether to let the Protective Brain or the Thoughtful Brain take control of the situation. When the prefrontal cortex, or Thoughtful Brain, is put in charge, we can focus, make good decisions, and learn.

While the Thoughtful Brain is what allows your child to choose what to focus on, the Protective Brain is busy trying to distract it, constantly demanding focus anytime something seems important or interesting. What makes this scenario particularly difficult for children is that the prefrontal cortex is not fully developed until our midtwenties. The Protective Brain has a very strong advantage in our kids. If we want to help them live a more balanced life, with the capacity for good decision making and focused attention, then we need to understand how challenging it is for their Thoughtful Brain to exert itself and learn how to encourage and support its development.*

How Are Emotions and Focus Connected?

As we've seen, in order for your child to improve his focus skills (and many other desirable traits), it's essential that he is able to access his prefrontal cortex. While many of the practices that we talk about in this book will help the Thoughtful Brain become stronger and more active in your child, there are many life circumstances that reinforce the natural advantage of the Protective Brain. Under conditions of stress, the Protective Brain is more likely to take control, and no amount of talking, begging, rationalizing, or demanding on your part will help your child transition to using his prefrontal cortex. You can help

---

* For a more complete discussion of the neurobiology of childhood, as well as parenting strategies to support healthy development, I strongly recommend Daniel Siegel and Tina Payne Bryson's *The Whole-Brain Child*.

strengthen the Thoughtful Brain of your child by helping him feel safe, calm, secure, and unconditionally accepted.

What Causes Stress in Children?

Stress is an epidemic in our society, and our children are not spared its impact. Kids themselves will often talk about feeling "stressed," but when we dig a little deeper into what they mean, what we often find is that stress is being used as a way to describe many different challenges and emotions. Described here are some common causes of stress in children, but there are many more, and if you tune in to your own child you will certainly find that he has his own unique combination of concerns that cause him stress.

Worry and Anxiety: Kids are often burdened with a tremendous amount of anxiety and little capacity to make meaningful changes to the things that cause the anxiety. Children are exposed to much of life's unpleasantness. For example, they are very aware of tensions between their parents, and they hear about violence and war on the news, yet often adults choose not to discuss these types of things with their kids, leaving children with no opportunity for perspective or capacity to ask questions. Some of the things that children worry about the most include concerns about their home and family, school success, social anxiety (Muris et al. 1998), fear of personal harm (Silverman, La Greca, and Wasserstein 1995), and not having enough time to get everything done.

Exhaustion: Our kids are chronically tired, and being tired leads to feeling overwhelmed. According to the 2004 Sleep in America poll, more then two-thirds of American children experience frequent problems getting enough sleep. Fatigue increases our sensitivity to negative emotions, reduces our tolerance of other people, and makes all of the things we need to do seem a little bit harder and a little more overwhelming. Even among children who get enough sleep, sensory overload can bring on a feeling of exhaustion. We live in a world that, from an evolutionary perspective, is filled with danger signs. Particularly in urban environments, children are exposed to near-constant bright lights, loud noises, and generally chaotic situations. The amount of stimuli that bombards our children at all times can become overwhelming to their nervous system, causing them to feel like they are always "on" and can't get any rest.

Feeling Disconnected: Human beings have a very high need for attachment. In children, this need is primary, and feeling lonely, disconnected, or not understood can have powerful consequences. The most important person for your child to feel connected to is you! When parents are tuned in to their children—connected to their emotions, sympathetic to their concerns, and responsive to their bids for affection—and create an environment where their child knows undoubtedly that he is loved and accepted regardless of his behavior, they create a foundation of safety and emotional stability that gives the child much greater resilience (Maté 2000). It's important to remember that you can love your child very much and still be so busy, distracted, or stressed out yourself that you don't provide him with the full strength of your attention.

Even before you begin the practices in this book, you can work to reduce the causes of stress in your child's life. Spend time engaging with your child fully and completely. Listen more attentively and proactively. Encourage him to talk with you about worries or concerns. Pay attention to his physical needs and be an advocate for getting him more rest, better nourishment, and opportunities to relax and restore. If you are your child's protector (not just of his body, but of his emotions and his sense of self), then the Protective Brain can take a break and the Thoughtful Brain will get stronger.

Emotional Intelligence

While nothing can eliminate all stress from anyone's life, learning to recognize the causes of stress, relating to emotions in a more productive way, and learning to work with your body to release stress can all help reduce its impact. In subsequent chapters we will discuss specific practices to reduce the impact of stress on the body and mind, and improve emotional intelligence.

In his 1995 book *Emotional Intelligence*, Daniel Goleman described emotional intelligence as "being able to motivate oneself and persist in the face of frustrations; to control impulse and to delay gratification; to regulate one's moods and keep distress from swamping the ability to think." I think of emotional intelligence as the ability to recognize and make sense of how you are feeling, so that your emotions don't become overwhelming and cause your Protective Brain to take over. When you understand how interrelated our emotions are with our focus and self-regulation skills, it becomes clear that emotional intelligence is crucial to the capacity to pay attention and learn.

Learning to Notice Your Mind

Supporting the development of your child's emotional intelligence will give her Thoughtful Brain support and strength. Calming and bringing balance to her emotions will allow the Protective Brain to relax its control. But keeping the Thoughtful Brain in charge also involves self-awareness skills that children can learn and practice. Improving the capacity to focus means learning to recognize when your mind is wandering and bring it back; and it means developing the capacity to filter irrelevant environmental stimuli and to let go of intrusive thoughts. These are skills that will be explored in the following chapters and that get easier with practice.

What Is My Child Experiencing?

While we've seen how challenging it can be for any child to remain focused and emotionally balanced and aware, for some—especially those struggling with ADHD, anxiety, or other diagnosed disorders, or those experiencing a particularly intense life event (such as a move, a new baby in the family, or a divorce)—that challenge can become substantially more difficult.

For children in these situations, life can be very confusing and overwhelming. The primary experience may be one of intense emotions, often with a limited self-understanding of where those emotions even came from. The impulsive and unpredictable behavior that is so common when the protective brain takes over can be intensely frustrating to parents, teachers, and even other children, causing the child to repeatedly feel isolated and misunderstood. These children often find themselves locked into the role of the troublemaker at school, with teachers mistakenly believing that the child is choosing when to focus and when to misbehave in some sort of deliberate action.

Because the Protective Brain of the child with a serious attention problem is often working at full strength, it is seeking all information that may signal danger or threat. This means the child is likely to be easily overstimulated and his sympathetic nervous system overactivated, with every noise, smell, and passing sight demanding attention, often in direct conflict with a parent or teacher talking. Filtering the tremendous amount of irrelevant stimuli that are a normal part of life—so that focus can be maintained on a single task, thought, or conversation—becomes a Herculean task.

These children are also typically exhausted, both physically and emotionally. The effort to relax is a constant struggle, as it is often only in doing and moving that they can find any degree of self-satisfaction. The intensity of their experiences and emotions is draining, and their exhaustion makes self-regulation even more difficult.

When a particularly sensitive child is raised in a stressful environment, the Protective Brain is called upon over and over again to defend the child from those stresses. Remember, the Protective Brain is already stronger and more dominant in childhood, and in a sensitive child it is even more responsive. The sensitive child doesn't need stress to be particularly traumatic or extreme in order to trigger the Protective Brain to take charge. And, when even a moderate level of stress is chronic, the brain gets trained to operate in the protective mode. Once the child's brain becomes hardwired in this way, the Protective Brain often exerts control even when there is no apparent stressor at the moment. This makes it much more difficult to access the Thoughtful Brain, and the symptoms of attention problems and impulsive behavior emerge. Changing these patterns of the brain is difficult, but possible, as we will explore in subsequent chapters.

What about ADHD?

ADHD is a developmental challenge that has caused a lot of controversy in the medical and education communities. There are three main features of ADHD, two of which are needed for a clinical diagnosis: poor attention skills, deficient impulse control, and hyperactivity. The hard part of diagnosing ADHD is that these traits exist in all of us, children and adults. Determining when the manifestation of these traits becomes a disorder needing treatment is a matter of degree and perspective.

What is undeniable is that there is a point for some children and adults when the challenges to daily life caused by these traits become substantial, and intervention becomes necessary in order to live a fulfilling, productive, and happy life. Gabor Maté, a noted physician and author of *Scattered: How Attention Deficit Disorder Originates and What You Can Do About It*, describes ADHD not as a "fixed, inherited brain disorder but as a physiological consequence of life in a particular environment, in a particular culture" (2000, 7), yet he also strongly supports the idea that ADHD is a very real physical manifestation of those consequences in the brain. From Dr. Maté's perspective (and I find his to be among the most thoughtful, carefully considered, and useful of the perspectives out there on the topic), ADHD develops in individuals when a combination of factors cause the structure of the brain to develop in a particular way. Human brains are unique in that they are relatively underdeveloped when we are born, and the majority of their growth happens during our lives, mainly during our childhood. This means that our life experiences have a direct impact on the shape of that growth. In children with serious attention difficulties, their life experiences have had the effect of essentially supercharging their Protective Brains.

What is it that determines if the traits of ADHD that are so common in our society become more seriously pronounced in one child and not another? According to Dr. Maté, it is the combination of a person that is particularly sensitive to stimulation (both sensory and emotional) and a chronically stressful infancy and childhood. Dr. Maté describes the latent potential to develop ADHD as similar to an allergy, but instead of the nervous system being hypersensitive to peanuts or bee stings, it's sensitive to overstimulation and stress (although children with ADHD are also more prone to colds, respiratory infections, ear infections, and allergies, lending support to the idea that their systems are more reactive in general). It's important to remember that this increased sensitivity is not a choice, it's a feature of the child's nervous system, and, in some ways, sensitivity is a positive thing, making the child more creative and capable of accessing the full range of human emotions.

What Can Help?

In the following chapters we will discuss how yoga and mindfulness practices can support children in the development of their Thoughtful Brain strength, and how these practices can work to restore emotional balance, increase focus, and generally support a more meaningful and fulfilling way of life. But even before you try a single activity in this book, remember that by helping your child reduce stress, making her feel unconditionally accepted and loved, and working to reduce your own anxiety and reactivity, you will be soothing her Protective Brain, creating space for her Thoughtful Brain to grow and working toward a greater capacity for self-regulation.

Also, on your most frustrating days, remember that your child is doing the best she can. And so are you. Be kind to yourself, be compassionate toward your child, and step by step, work to create a home environment that will let you both become the best versions of yourselves.

chapter 2

Explore

The word "yoga" has come to represent many different things to people in our culture. For some, it signifies an exercise program, for others a meditative form of stress relief or a therapeutic modality for healing from an injury. Some people use the word "yoga" as a way of describing someone they see as having a particular set of social or political values, as in "she's such a yoga person" or "I'm not a yoga person." In this chapter, we will explore what the traditions of yoga and mindfulness have to offer us as parents and teachers, as well as how these practices can help our children access the very best aspects of themselves.

What Is Yoga?

"*Yoga chitta vritti nirodha*" is a phrase from the *Yoga Sutras*, a text widely attributed to the sage Patanjali, written more than two thousand years ago. The *Yoga Sutras* are in many ways the defining text of the tradition of yoga (though Patanjali didn't invent yoga, he just wrote down the principles). The exact translation of this Sanskrit phrase varies, but the most common is "Yoga is the cessation of fluctuations in the mind." Another translation that I love is "Yoga is the uniting of consciousness in the heart" (Devi 2007, 17). When you think about these traditional definitions of yoga, it's immediately apparent that we are talking about something much bigger than an exercise program.

The yoga practice is rooted in a philosophical tradition that sees human suffering as the result of our own minds constantly thinking about the past, projecting into the future, worrying about things that may never happen, blaming ourselves for things that couldn't be helped, and otherwise remaining stuck in a mental state that is unrelated to the truth of the present moment. Yoga is designed to be a path toward a place of integration where your mind, your heart, and your body are healthy, connected to each other, and tuned in to the world around you. It's designed to be a path toward the very best version of yourself. And the happiest version of yourself.

While we often talk about practicing yoga, or doing yoga, or going to yoga class, the most appropriate use of the word "yoga" is as the end goal. When we do all of these things we are working to reach a state of Yoga where we are fully whole, integrated within ourselves, and connected mindfully and meaningfully to the world around us. When you recognize that Yoga is the goal, it's easy to see that there are many possible paths to achieving it. Within the yoga tradition there are a wide variety of paths, or practices, that can bring a person to this state of integration. The particular path that has become most familiar in the Western world, and a path that is particularly well suited to sharing with children, is the path of *ashtanga yoga*, or the Eight-Limbed Path.

While yoga is a traditional practice thousands of years old, it has been evolving over time to meet the needs of a changing environment, and it is also in some ways uniquely suited for modern life. The *ashtanga* path of yoga addresses many of the most profound internal challenges of our lives and our children's lives: overwhelming stress, poor physical health, overstimulation, and disconnection.

Mindfulness and the Eight-Limbed Path

While yoga has been evolving for thousands of years, so has a similar tradition called mindfulness. *Mindfulness meditation* is a specific type of meditation, the goal of which is nonjudgmental moment-to-moment awareness of the present. This definition was made popular by Jon Kabat-Zinn, the founding director of the Stress Reduction Clinic and the Center for Mindfulness in Medicine, Health Care, and Society at the University of Massachusetts Medical School. Kabat-Zinn studied the Buddhist tradition of mindfulness meditation, combined it with Western science, and presented it in a secular format to create the Mindfulness-Based Stress-Reduction Program (MBSR), which is used in medical settings around the world. The MBSR program has become one of the most studied forms of meditation in the West, with tremendously positive outcomes for a wide variety of populations. The goal of MBSR, and mindfulness meditation in general, is to reduce stress, suffering, and even the experience of pain through an increased awareness of the present moment. By seeing things as they really are and becoming capable of acting with that awareness, we can reduce reactivity and impulsiveness and live life with more intention.

If this sounds familiar, it's because the goals of mindfulness and the goals of yoga are virtually identical. While mindfulness meditation has its own traditions, practices, and teachings, mindfulness is also a fundamental part of the *ashtanga* yoga path, and the *ashtanga* yoga path is a particularly clear and effective route toward mindfulness. As we've seen in our earlier discussion, our bodies, our minds, and even our relationships with others are all inextricably connected. The Eight-Limbed Path provides a practice that honors these interconnections. It offers a systematic approach with a road map accessible to anyone, at any stage of life.

So what are these eight limbs we keep talking about? The eight limbs are aspects of the yoga practice that are all equally important. They support each other and work together to guide us toward a state of Yoga. They are presented here in the traditional order that they appear in in the *Yoga Sutras*, but they don't have to be practiced or taught in this particular order. While the aspects of the practice are called limbs, they may be better thought of as a circle or a spiral. Regardless of which one you start with, if you continue to practice you will find yourself moving through them all at ever higher levels of self-awareness, wellness, and peace.

The Yamas

The first limb is known as the *yamas*, which are often thought of as guidelines for interacting with the world and are the building blocks of your practice. Nischala Joy Devi, a renowned yoga teacher and author of *The Healing Path of Yoga*, as well as an excellent translation of the *Yoga Sutras*, defines *yamas* as "reflection of our true nature." The translations of the *yamas* and *niyamas* that follow are hers (Devi 2007, 167):

- *Ahimsa*: "reverence, love, and compassion for all"

- *Satya*: "truthfulness and integrity"

- *Astheya*: "generosity and honesty"

- *Brahmacharya*: "balance and moderation of the vital life force"

- *Aparigraha*: "awareness of abundance, fulfillment"

Ahimsa ("reverence, love, and compassion for all") is considered the most fundamental of the *yamas*. If there is ever a conflict between, for example, truthfulness and love and compassion, *ahimsa* is considered the higher calling. Don't forget the importance of treating yourself with reverence, love, and compassion as well!

The Niyamas

As the *yamas* describe ways to interact with the world, the *niyamas* describe ways to foster your own inner peace and harmony.

- *Saucha*: "simplicity"

- *Santosha*: "contentment"

- *Tapas*: "zeal and sincerity"

- *Swadyaya*: "study and introspection"

- *Iswara Pranidhana*: "wholehearted dedication"

The *niyama* of *iswara pranidhana* can be confusing. When the sutras encourage wholehearted dedication, what are they suggesting we dedicate ourselves to? Yoga is a practice of many paths, and there is no one right object of dedication, such as in a religion. The suggestion of *iswara pranidhana* is to open your heart to a universe that is larger than yourself—to make your own decisions about what moves your spirit, whether it is a symbol of divinity, an element of nature, a philosophy, or a cause—and to allow dedication to those things to fill your heart and connect you to something universal and inspiring.

Asana — a steady & comfortable seat

Asana is the third limb of the yoga path and typically the one that most people are familiar with. It is the movement, the postures, the physical practice. Often people think that the translation of "asana" is "yoga pose," but the sutra that describes asana is "*sthira sukham asanam*." The translation of the words "*sthira*" and "*sukham*" are "effortless" and "a state of comfort or joy," respectively. One useful translation of "asana" is "a steady and comfortable seat."

Usually, people don't think of yoga poses in terms like "comfortable" and "joyful," but the goal of the asana practice is not to bend and twist our bodies into awkward and uncomfortable positions. The yoga path values the physical practice of our moving bodies for several reasons, and with several goals in mind. One is to reduce discomfort and distraction caused by the physical body. When asana is practiced regularly, the body becomes healthier, stronger, more flexible, and overall a nicer place for your spirit to live. When your body has greater health and less discomfort, your mind can be much clearer and more open for the meditation practices that are to come (and for the learning and development of childhood).

Another goal of the asana practice, and one we will talk about in the activities sections of this book, is to learn more about yourself through the movement. When we practice asana, we create all kinds of circumstances that we then have thoughts, feelings, and reactions to. Learning to notice how your body and your mind are handling these different situations, both the challenging ones and the ones that feel good, can teach you a tremendous amount about yourself and help you learn to see past your initial reaction to things (and strengthen your Thoughtful Brain in the process). Practicing challenging asana in a safe environment gives you and your child a chance to practice getting comfortable, feeling secure, and maybe even finding some joy in situations that are not easy.

Pranayama

[handwritten: ✦ — very important — to reduce anxiety, good "concentration"]

The fourth limb of *ashtanga* yoga, *pranayama*, is the "enhancement and guidance of prana, or energy." Our energetic life force is primarily maintained and manipulated by our breath. When our energetic state changes, for example, when we are resting or scared or exercising, our breath changes in response. The reverse is also true. When we change our breath, we can change our energetic state, encouraging increased energy or an increased sense of calm. When we practice *pranayama*, we practice deliberately changing the pace, rhythm, and pattern of our breath in an effort to bring our energy into greater balance, soothe our nervous system, and use our life force most effectively.

Pratyahara

[handwritten: dharana, dhyana]

The fifth limb is *pratyahara*: the drawing inward of our senses and the beginning of the practice of meditation (which we will discuss more in the following two limbs, *dharana* and *dhyana*). Usually, we use our senses to understand the outside world. We see and smell and taste and hear and touch, and as we do so we gather information about our environment and about other people. These senses of ours are very good at what they do and are an essential part of life, but they can also be tremendously distracting, keeping our attention and awareness riveted outside of ourselves. The practice of *pratyahara* teaches us to draw our senses close, turning them away from the stimulation of the outside world and using them to gather information about, and better understand, ourselves.

Dharana and Dhyana

As we move into the practice of *dharana* ("contemplation" or "single-pointed focus"), we are starting on a continuum of meditation experience. From *pratyahara*, we develop a greater capacity to turn inward and reduce the distractions of sensory experiences. This practice makes *dharana* substantially more accessible. *Dhyana*, our next limb, is a natural continuation of *dharana*, as it is just a sustained and more effortless state of *dhyana*.

In the practice of single-pointed focus, we train our minds to stay present and connected to one thing. The object of connection is just a tool to help with the practice and can be anything, from our breath to an object that we look at, such as a candle, to a mantra or saying that we repeat internally. During this practice, it is entirely natural for the mind to wander away from the chosen object over and over again. The whole point of practicing *dharana* is to notice when the mind wanders and get in the habit of bringing it back to the object of focus.

As we practice *dharana*, the length of time that awareness stays connected to the object of focus will become longer, and the times the mind wanders and must be brought back will become fewer. At some undefined point in this practice, when the sustaining of attention becomes effortless and prolonged, we slip from the practice of *dharana* into the state of *dhyana*, or meditation.

Samadhi

The culmination of all of these practices is leading us toward a state of what is called in Sanskrit "*samadhi*." The eighth limb, *samadhi* has been translated in many different ways, often as "bliss" or "union with a universal energy." Many teachers say that *samadhi* cannot be explained, only experienced, but I think it is helpful to have some sense of where we are headed with all of this effort we've put into our yoga practice. I think of *samadhi* as a state of being where the practices of the first seven limbs of yoga have created an ability for us to be mindfully present to every moment of our lives. Tuned in to our experiences, we can be truly connected to the world around us. As our minds learn to live in the present, we are freed of the suffering that ruminating on the past and worrying about the future often bring.

The Five Elements of Little Flower Yoga

The LFY method of teaching yoga to children is rooted in the *ashtanga* yoga path, but in an effort to make the practice simpler and more appropriate for children, the eight limbs have been distilled into five elements.

Connect

Connect activities help children tune in and make sense of their experiences. They are practices that are used to develop mindful awareness of both the external world and the internal emotional state. The guiding principles of the *yamas* and *niyamas* have been considered in our Connect activities, and many of them also incorporate the practice of *pratyahara* (drawing inward of the senses).

Breathe

The breath is one of the most powerful tools for self-regulation. Breathe activities, based in traditional practices, help children learn to reduce anxiety, stabilize energy, and create a sense of safety and peace in the body.

Move

Move activities are based on asana practices that help children maintain a state of alert engagement, whereby hyperactive behavior is minimized but the child still feels strong and energetic.

Focus

The Focus activities in this program, rooted in *dharana* practices, provide deliberate meditations that teach children how to apply their focus in a step-by-step way, allowing for progressive improvement and experiences of success.

Relax

The final element of our program, Relax, gives children tools for rest, relaxation, and restoration. Exhaustion is common in children, and we know that being tired makes everything else, including paying attention, much harder. These activities, which are drawn from both asana and *dharana* practices, teach ways to rejuvenate, even when you aren't sleeping.

Each one of these elements serves as the basis for chapters 4 through 8. While the elements have benefits on their own, like the limbs of *ashtanga* yoga they only provide the richest experience and strongest impact in combination.

How Do We Know That Yoga Works?

While the efficacy of yoga is supported by thousands of years of tradition and wisdom passed from teacher to student, yoga has also been the subject of an increasing amount of research as it has become more popular in the West. Science now supports many of the benefits traditionally associated with yoga practice, including decreased stress and increased physical and emotional wellness. Recent advances in neuroscience confirm that contemplative practices, such as yoga and meditation, can change the physical structure of the brain, effectively training it to work in more positive and productive ways.

Increasing Attention

Yoga practice has traditionally been associated with an increased capacity for sustaining attention. One of the eight limbs, *dharana*, is dedicated to concentration, and aspects of breathwork and movement support it. This has been an interesting area of study for researchers, who are beginning to confirm this traditional knowledge. In one study, students who practiced mindful breathing reported that they were better able to focus, relax, reduce anxiety before taking a test, make better decisions when in conflict, and redirect their attention when off task (Napoli, Drech, and Holley 2005). A 2004 study published in the *Journal of Attention Disorders* found a reduction in restlessness, impulsivity, and inattentiveness specifically in boys with ADHD after twenty weeks of weekly yoga sessions (Jensen and Kenny 2004). In a 2011 study, Adele Diamond, a leader in the field of cognitive neuroscience, found that yoga (particularly an approach that addressed both physical practice and social and emotional development) was among practices that improved executive function in four- to twelve-year-olds. "Executive function" refers to the "set of cognitive functions involved in the top-down control of behavior" (Diamond and Lee 2011). It is what allows us to regulate our behavior, make good decisions, control our impulses, and selectively apply our attention. Improvements in executive function mean that the Thoughtful Brain is getting stronger.

Studies on mindfulness and meditation have also shown promising results in both children and adults. Several years' worth of very interesting work led by Antoine Lutz and Richard Davidson has shown that meditators, even beginners, had increased activation in regions of their brains needed for controlling attention. One of their most recent studies has additionally shown that extremely experienced meditators had less brain activation

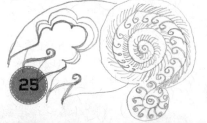
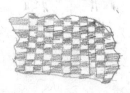

while also performing attention-related tasks better, attesting that meditation actually made paying attention easier for the brain (Slagter, Davidson, and Lutz 2011). While this work was done on adults, other studies on children support similar ideas. In 2010, Randye Semple, a clinical psychologist at the University of Southern California, found that participants in a mindfulness-based cognitive therapy program for children had reduced attention problems and that these improvements were maintained for at least three months following the intervention (Semple et al. 2010).

Preliminary research on mindfulness introduced in a school setting suggests that the practice is particularly beneficial for children with executive function difficulties, with students showing increased executive function, specifically working memory, as well as planning and organizational skills (Flook et al. 2010) and inhibitory control (a measure of attention) (Oberle et al. 2012). In a review of current research, Kelly McGonigal (2012), a teacher of psychology, yoga, and meditation at Stanford University, discusses how concentration meditation "makes you better at focusing on something specific while ignoring distractions" and "can make you more capable of noticing what is happening around you."

Creating Greater Emotional Balance

As we saw in our discussion in chapter 1, improved attention and emotional balance are intimately connected to one another. One of the benefits of yoga that practitioners often notice early on in their experience is a decreased reactivity to frustrating stimuli and an increased sense of perspective and overall well-being. The path of yoga is meant to be a way to reduce the suffering created by our own minds, and bringing balance to our emotions is an integral part of this process.

Several recent studies have supported these traditional teachings. In 2009, the *Journal of Alternative Therapies in Health and Medicine* published a pilot study of fourth- and fifth-grade students in New York who attended an after-school yoga class once a week for twelve weeks. After just twelve yoga sessions, the children who participated showed increased well-being and enhanced self-worth, and fewer negative behaviors were reported in response to stress (Berger, Silver, and Stein 2009). Another study of young adults in 2004 found a reduction in symptoms among people with mild depression after just five weeks of yoga practice (Woolery et al. 2004).

Other research looking at more specific aspects of the practice has shown positive impact on emotional balance as well. Among teens and young adults, focused breathing has been shown to increase tolerance for remaining in contact with unpredictable

[handwritten margin notes: children; Yoga -12 weeks; 12 times; focusing attention]

negative stimuli (Arch and Craske 2006), and focusing attention and awareness on a single point (as in the practice of *dharana*) has been found to promote a relaxation response (Roeser and Peck 2009). Mindfulness meditation intervention has been shown to have a positive impact on problematic responses to stress in children including rumination, intrusive thoughts, and emotional arousal (Mendelson et al. 2010).

As more researchers become interested in the impact of yoga and meditation, the findings have become increasingly more complex and interesting. A 2009 study led by Eileen Luders from the UCLA School of Medicine showed that meditators had more gray matter in the prefrontal cortex, responsible for attention, emotional regulation, and mental flexibility. More recent work out of UCLA has found an increase in gyrification, or folding of the cortex, in meditators. These folds are thought to allow the brain to process information more effectively. This study (Luders et al. 2012) found a direct link between number of years of meditation and amount of folding. Another 2012 study (Froeliger, Garland, and McClernon) looked at a yoga practices including movement, breathwork, and meditation. It found that practitioners had more gray matter in frontal, limbic, temporal, occipital, and cerebellar regions of the brain, and that increased gray matter was positively correlated with duration of the yoga practice. This same study found that yoga practitioners reported significantly fewer cognitive failures (such as forgetting where something was left, getting distracted, having trouble making decisions, etc.).

Recent work done by Philippe Goldin, a research scientist in the psychology department at Stanford University, has shown that mindfulness meditation can actually change the way the brain responds to negative thoughts, and that practitioners show a decrease in gray matter density in the amygdala (Goldin, Ramel, and Gross 2009). In the same 2012 article mentioned earlier, Kelly McGonigal notes that "previous research had revealed that trauma and chronic stress can enlarge the amygdala and make it more reactive and more connected to other areas of the brain, leading to greater stress and anxiety. This study is one of the first documented cases showing change occurring in the opposite direction—with the brain instead becoming less reactive and more resilient." While these researchers have been looking at the impact of meditation on the brains of adults (and more research is needed to fully understand the impact of these practices on the developing minds of children), the findings are significant, compelling, and extremely encouraging.

chapter 3

Get Started

The next five chapters of this book are filled with activities for you to share with your child. But before you get started there are some things that you'll want to keep in mind, and some preparations to make.

Guiding Principles for Sharing Yoga with Your Child

The following guidelines are essential principles that are more important than any of the individual activities. They should remind you of what is important as you undertake this work with your child. And if you find yourself forgetting to follow them, try to take a step back, evaluate your own emotions, and find some time for your personal practice.

Your child is more important than the yoga. Your child is an individual, and her needs and feelings must come first. This may seem obvious, but adults can get so wrapped up in our desire to teach or share an activity that we forget to stay connected to the child's experience. Pay attention to how your child is receiving the activity, and if she needs to slow down, start over, or even do something completely different on that day, then be sensitive to those needs.

Participation needs to be a choice. Children generally don't benefit much from activities that they participate in under duress. Think about ways to engage your child in the activities, and start with the ones that you think will be most interesting to him. Make connections between the activities and the things that your child cares about in his life. Even if your child resists participation at first, you can still provide information and model the activities—he will absorb what you are doing and saying. Continue to set aside time to practice the activities during the day, and continually invite your child to participate with you.

If something doesn't feel right, stop. A big part of yoga is learning to meet your own needs and recognize your own boundaries. Make sure you tell your child early and often that if something hurts, feels uncomfortable, or just doesn't feel right, that she can stop. It's always appropriate in yoga to take a rest, slow down, or decide to do something different. Support these choices and encourage your child to always share how she is feeling.

A good outcome is not always the one you expected. When you begin an activity or a conversation with your child, you may have a particular outcome in mind. It's easy to try to measure success, both for your child and for yourself as a parent, against how close your child comes to this outcome. But what happens so often is that your child's mind isn't working the same way yours is, and if you allow him to have some creative freedom and some mental space, the outcome you get may be one that you had never even considered. Try to let go of your preconceptions, and remember that a good result is not necessarily the same one that you were planning.

Prioritize quality of experience over quantity of activities. Don't rush! The activities in this book are not meant to be accomplished one after the other like a checklist of lessons. Take your time, and encourage your child to fully explore each of the activities. If something is very compelling to your child, continue to practice it and don't feel like you are somehow wasting your time on something she has already "learned." As long as she is engaged by the experience, she is still acquiring valuable skills from it. Every child will have a unique path through these activities, and it's always more important that she have a complete and positive experience than get through them all in any particular time frame (or ever!). Remember, there is nothing to accomplish here, only things to practice.

Make sure your child experiences more successes than challenges. You want to inspire confidence in your child, but sometimes it's easy to focus so much on challenging our kids that we forget how important it is to nurture their spirits. Parents have a tremendous impact on their children's beliefs about their own competence and capacity for achievement. When children don't believe that success is possible for them, learned helplessness can set in, whereby children feel that it is impossible for them to succeed, so they stop trying. It is your job to make sure that your child has the opportunity to experience many more successes then failures. This doesn't mean that you shouldn't challenge him and teach him to work toward a difficult goal, but if you know you are about to work on something that might be frustrating, make sure to bracket that experience with activities that you know he can feel good about.

Your attitude changes everything. The attitude that you approach these practices with will make a huge difference in your child's experience. If you embrace the activities with a spirit of curiosity, playfulness, and exploration, your child will be much more likely to do the same. As you practice and learn together, remember that these things are new, and what your child needs is compassion, acceptance, and support in order to feel positive about them. Try to use this time together to break out of any previously established negative patterns of interaction. Make sure your child knows that you are on her side. Take a look at the suggestions in chapter 10 for maintaining positive communication with your child, and check out some of the recommended additional reading on the topic.

Making Space for Yoga

Life is busy and full, and creating space for something new can be challenging. While yoga and mindfulness can be practiced as an integral part of daily life, when you and your child are first exploring these activities you will have to create space in your home, space in your schedule, and even space in your own mind and emotions.

Taking the time to prepare carefully will set the stage for a successful experience. When you show your child that something is worth creating space for, rather than just being squeezed in between all the busyness, it gives that thing value and changes the way he perceives it. You want your child to see that you are creating space in your life for yoga, and, more important, space in your life for him!

Physical Space

When you start practicing yoga with your child, it is important to choose an area of your home that will support her experience. Choose someplace quiet where you are not likely to be interrupted or disturbed. A room where you can close the door is best. The place you choose to practice should feel very safe to both of you and ideally should remain the same for each session.

While rooms for children often contain a large amount of stimulating things such as pictures, colorful objects, mirrors, and lots of books, the best space in which to practice yoga (especially if you are struggling with focus and attention) is one that is very clean, with limited distractions. Your child will benefit from a space where you've worked to reduce clutter and visual noise. If the scenery outside the window is natural and calm (such as a view of trees or water), go ahead and leave the shades open, but if you can see the street or neighbor's children playing outside, close the blinds. Try to choose a space without mirrors, and if there is one in the room cover it with a sheet. It's a great idea to choose a space where you have the option to dim the lights, or if that isn't possible bring a scarf or two to lay over the lamps when needed.

If you are setting up your yoga space in a room that is regularly used by your child for another purpose, think about what you can do to make it feel more special for your yoga practice time. Maybe you can set up a diffuser to fill the room with a scent that your child enjoys (lavender or vanilla often work well for kids), or bring a special object to place in front of you during your practice. Natural objects that connect to the seasons often can work for this. For example, set up a beautiful vase of flowers in the spring and summer, choose a selection of leaves and pinecones in the fall, and plant a tiny evergreen tree in a pot for the winter. Don't go overboard and load up your clean, simple space with lots of stimuli—just choose one thing that will help make the space feel special, and keep it consistent.

Simple Space & with nature & less stimuli

Yoga Mats. Singing Bowl (O) Eye Pillow

Mats and Materials

You will definitely want to use yoga mats for both you and your child during these activities, even if your space is carpeted. Mats provide grounding and structure. They give each of you personal space with clear boundaries and a sense of having a home base. Many children get quite attached to their yoga mat. It feels like their own safe space. For this reason I don't recommend using a mat that you have around the house or one that is shared by other family members. If it is at all possible, purchase a yoga mat specifically for your child, ideally with his input. If you can do this in a store, let your child feel the mats and choose one that he likes. If you are ordering a mat online, let him choose the color. Consider purchasing a mat made of natural rubber, which will be a healthier surface for your child to spend time on.

There are a few other materials that you may consider assembling for your yoga space. You won't need all of them for each session, but having them close by will make it easier to change course if your plan for the day doesn't match your child's needs.

Singing Bowl: A singing bowl is a small metal bowl that comes with a wooden striker and can be rung much like a bell. Using a singing bowl for mindful listening practices is very effective. The fact that it is a unique object that your child is not used to seeing in her daily life makes it feel more special and interesting. The resonance of the bowl makes it more appealing to listen to than a simple bell, with a richer sound that lasts longer. You can often find singing bowls for sale at yoga studios, and a quick Internet search will also offer you plenty of options.

Eye Pillow: A small eye pillow is a wonderful thing to use during restorative and relaxing activities, particularly if your child struggles to keep his eyes closed and his body still. The gentle weight of an eye pillow is very soothing and encourages deeper relaxation.

Several Firm Blankets: There may be times during yoga poses that you or your child will want some extra support under hips, knees, back, or head. Having some blankets around that you can fold into various shapes and sizes is the simplest way to meet this need. Blankets that are very soft or fluffy don't work as well as simple thin ones do.

Journal or Notebook, Drawing Paper, and Colored Pencils or Crayons: Some activities call for journaling or drawing specifically, and even when they don't it's a great idea to have these materials available to your child anytime she wants to use them to process or reflect during or after her yoga practice.

Firm Blankets for support.
Socks.

What to Wear

You don't need to purchase special clothes for yoga! You and your child should both wear something comfortable that you can move freely in. Remember that you'll be putting your body in all different shapes, so wear something that will stay put and not make you feel uncomfortable if you are bending or stretching.

Practicing yoga barefoot is a good idea, because you will be able to balance better and avoid slipping. If you are worried about your feet getting cold, bring some socks with you to your space to wear during seated or reclining activities.

Space in Time

Finding time in your day and in your child's day to establish a regular practice can be challenging. It is important to make time for consistent, scheduled sessions, as well as finding ways to work yoga and mindfulness activities into your daily life. It is more important to make time for regular, frequent sessions than it is to make your sessions very long.

Establishing a Routine

Give some thought to both your child's schedule and your own, and decide on a time that you can dedicate to your yoga practice at least once per week. If you can find two or three times per week that is even better. Start with an amount of time that feels manageable for your family. Even fifteen or twenty minutes on a consistent basis will be great. Some people find that one longer session during the weekend plus one or two shorter fifteen- to twenty-minute sessions during the week provides a nice balance.

Once you've decided on your schedule, do your best not to change it. Establishing a routine will help make these practices a stabilizing and supportive force in your child's life. Knowing that he can count on this time and that you've prioritized it will mean a lot to your child (even if it seems like he would rather do something else); rescheduling his practice will make it feel less important. Because this consistency really matters, make sure that the schedule you choose is manageable. You can always add to it later.

Once you've established your regularly scheduled yoga time, you can start thinking about how you want to incorporate the activities from the next five chapters into that space. My recommendation is to stay simple and open-minded, and not try to plan very far in advance. As we discussed in the previous chapter, the LFY program consists of five elements—Connect, Breathe, Move, Focus, and Relax. Try to expose your child to activities from each element during the course of the week. Depending on how you have arranged your schedule, that may mean doing just one activity on any given day, which is completely fine. You do not have to teach the activities in the order that they appear in this book. Go ahead and mix and match based on what you think will work for your child on any particular day.

Let your child's interest drive the pace at which you add new activities. It makes sense to repeat practices that your child enjoys and shows engagement with. Allow him to have a progressively more in-depth experience. Feel confident that as long as he is engaged by the activity, he is still learning from it. Don't be in a rush to add new activities if things are feeling good.

Opening and Closing Rituals

Consider making a simple opening and closing ritual part of your regularly scheduled practice sessions. These rituals will provide simple transitions for both you and your child, allowing you to start your practice time in a more centered way and honoring the work you've done before heading back out into your family life.

An opening ritual that we use in many LFY classes is to gently ring a singing bowl one time, listen for the whole sound to finish, and then practice a few rounds of Heart and Belly Breath (see chapter 5). This only takes a minute or two, but it creates an energetic shift that supports all of the work you are about to do.

Your closing ritual should also be simple. A traditional way to end a yoga class is to bring your hands to your heart and say *"Namaste"* to each other. This is a lovely Sanskrit word that can be translated as "the light inside of me bows to the light inside of you." Another option is a Singing Bowl Send-Out. In this activity, you and your child would each take a turn holding the singing bowl up to your heart, imagining filling that bowl with love, and then ringing it one time to send all that love out to someone who needs it.

Feel free to make up your own opening and closing rituals with your child. The important thing is that they are simple, feel good, and create the energetic effect that you are looking for.

Daily Life Integration

In addition to your scheduled yoga time, you will want to open your life to the creation of mindful moments. Once your child begins to get comfortable with the practices, start looking for ways to incorporate them into her day-to-day experience, even for just a minute or two at a time. Each activity described in the following chapters includes suggestions for daily practice. If your child enjoys an activity during your yoga time, make sure you talk with her about these options.

Emotional Space

Once you've created a physical space in your home and space in your schedule, it can be easy to overlook the need for you as a parent to create some emotional space for the work you are about to undertake. Yoga is a nurturing and fulfilling practice, but it also can contain unexpected challenges and frustrations. Sharing yoga with your child is bound to have you questioning your assumptions, rethinking some ideas, and struggling with your own emotions. Your personal preparation will make a tremendous difference in the experience of your child, both during these practices and in everyday life.

Make sure that you take time for yourself and commit to your own personal practice. Your practice can look very different from your child's. Remember that when you take care of yourself, it not only makes you better able to care for your child, it also provides him with a powerful example of self-care.

What to Expect from the Following Chapters

The next five chapters are broken down into each of the five LFY elements and will provide you with activities to share with your child. In each chapter you'll find an introduction that gives you more detailed information about the element, along with some suggestions for teaching the activities. The activities themselves are offered with simple step-by-step instructions. After the instructions, you'll find three short paragraphs—follow-up, challenges, and daily practice.

The *follow-up* section after each activity will give you some thoughts for expanding the experience and providing your child with extra support. In *challenges* we discuss common struggles that kids experience in the activity, along with ways to help. The *daily practice* paragraph will offer you some thoughts on how to integrate the activity into your child's day-to-day life.

It is important that you practice these activities yourself before teaching them to your child. You should know how the activities feel, what emotions they might bring up, and what sensations they produce. When you share the activities with your child, you want to be able to understand his experience and give him guidance based on a true knowledge of what you are asking of him. You might even find that some of the activities you think are just for your child become a favorite part of your own personal practice!

Dive In

You will never be 100 percent prepared for this undertaking. Don't be afraid to just dive in and get started sharing yoga and mindfulness with your child. Make sure you read and practice the whole activity that you are about to share, but don't worry if you haven't read this whole book! As long as you approach the work (and your child) with love, compassion, and a sense of playful curiosity, you will be providing a positive experience that helps her become the best version of herself.

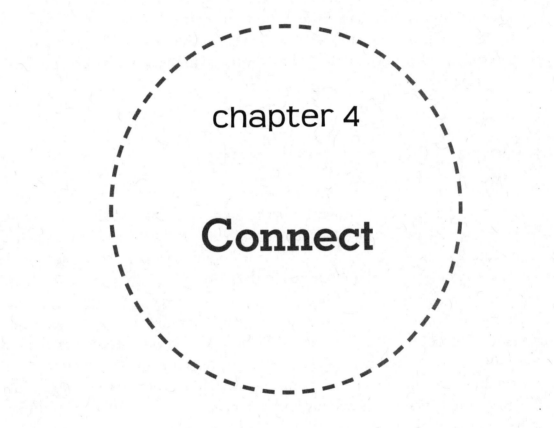

chapter 4

Connect

When your child is struggling to maintain focus, a challenging aspect of the problem is often a persistent feeling of being disconnected from others and from the present moment. Your child may find that his mind is always wandering, sometimes without him even being aware of it. It can be startling for a child to suddenly realize that he has missed an important part of a conversation, or that his teacher has been calling his name and he didn't hear it until the third or fourth call. We've all had times when we feel fragmented, ineffective, and overwhelmed—when we can't remember what we were thinking about, or realize we are listening to someone talk but have no idea what he or she just said. The stimulation of modern life increases these moments, and for many children this sense of disconnection is frequent and frustrating.

In this chapter we will explore activities that can help reorient your child to his present-moment experience, as well as train the mind to stay tuned in to what is happening physically, mentally, and emotionally.

Why Does Connecting Matter?

The inability to stay connected to present-moment experiences has an impact on many areas of your child's life. In social settings it may be hard for her to connect with friends as she struggles to maintain conversation; she may often miss the pauses and nonverbal cues that indicate it's her—or someone else's—turn to participate. As a result, friends might think she is tuning out or not interested in them.

In academic settings, the refrain of *pay attention* is likely to be something your child hears all day. You may have heard teachers tell you that your child is so smart and could be so successful in school if only she would "apply herself." We will discuss strategies in later chapters that can help your child focus on what she is trying to learn (and that can help you communicate with her teachers), but first we need to recognize that if your child is expending all of her energy on simply trying to remain present and aware (and even awake) in her classroom, then she may not have much mental energy left for learning.

The emotional consequences of this sense of disconnection can vary substantially from child to child. When so many things are pulling at your child's attention, the nervous system never gets a chance to rest. Your child isn't getting any downtime. This can lead to an increase in anxiety and a sense of constant worry. Noted physician Gabor Maté (2000) describes the feeling as being akin to always worrying that you have something that you are supposed to be doing but never being able to remember what it is.

This frenetic feeling is like a constant companion that serves to distract children away from the other emotions that they are experiencing. This overlay of anxiety colors their emotions, heightening some and damping others. In this context, it can be very hard for your child to make meaningful decisions and take appropriate actions, because what she is experiencing emotionally is not necessarily connected to the reality of the present moment.

Connecting to External and Internal Experiences

This chapter explores activities that help your child tune in to both the external environment, and the emotional landscape of internal experience. Both types of connection are crucial for experiencing the richness of life and navigating successfully through it. Becoming more aware of your external experiences, and practicing staying connected to those experiences, will, over time, contribute to your capacity to more accurately recognize your inner emotional experience and lessen the stress and anxiety that come from constantly wrapping your mind around the past, present, and future all at once.

The Practices

The following activities will help your child connect to what is around him and tune in to the most essential aspects of his experience. Practicing these activities will develop a habit of slowing down, increasing awareness, and experiencing life in a more complete way.

Don't worry about your child understanding the activities in a cerebral way. Instead just let him actually have the experience. When we practice mindfulness we are working on rewiring the brain. The experience itself does the work. It's not important for the child to *get it* or make some sort of larger connection to his life. Just allow the activities to unfold and, through repetition, become a part of your child's life.

Keep in mind that while some of these activities may seem simple, they will be a challenge for any child. It is your job to cultivate a sense of exploration and playfulness during these practices. Your child should not feel any pressure or judgment. You will want to internalize the idea that there is no one right way to practice mindfulness and yoga. The activities are all experiences and explorations. The success is in the trying, and each repetition strengthens the mind and contributes to developing a habit of awareness.

It is very useful to try these practices yourself before introducing them to your child so that you can better understand the experience and anticipate your child's challenges and questions.

Connecting with Life Experiences

The first three activities in this chapter—Layers of Sound, Walking Meditation, and Mindful Eating—are about learning to slow down and experience the complete fullness of daily life. Staying connected to what is happening in the present is the first step toward developing more control over your attention.

CONNECT:
LAYERS OF SOUND

Breath → far sound → Silence → Few min → listen
(Near Sound) (hear ur body)
Silence in between

Layers of Sound

This mindful listening practice asks your child to explore what she can hear around her in an intentional way. Our hearing is so sensitive. We don't have any way to block out sound the way we can close our eyes to reduce what we see. All of the sounds around us are competing for our attention all of the time. Learning to attune our hearing to the sounds that are most important at the moment is a life skill that children are called upon to exercise from the moment they enter school.

1. First, find a still and comfortable position for your body. It's fine to sit in a chair or lean against the wall. The most important thing is that you are comfortable enough to be still for just a few minutes. It may be helpful to close your eyes for this activity. If it doesn't feel good to close your eyes, let them rest on the ground right in front of you.

2. Now that you are still and comfortable, take a full breath or two to help you get ready for what's going to come next.

3. The first sounds that we are going to listen for are those that are far away from us. Open your ears as wide as you can make them, and imagine stretching your hearing way out beyond the room you are sitting in, and maybe even beyond the house that room is in, all the way to the outdoors. Listen carefully and find the farthest away sounds that you can hear.

4. When you start hearing sounds, don't worry about identifying the sound or figuring out what is making the sound. Just notice it exactly as it is. (Give the child a few minutes of silence here.)

5. Now that you have heard the farthest away sounds you can find, bring your hearing in a little bit closer, and find the sounds that are in this house. Again, don't worry about figuring out what is making the sounds, just listen for them.

6. Next we are going to bring our hearing even closer, to find the sounds that are in this room. Reach your hearing into each corner of the room and see what sounds you can find.

7. After you have found all of the sounds in the room, we are going to bring our hearing to the closest place of all—our own bodies.

8. Pull your hearing all the way to your body. Pull it out of the room and turn it to the sounds that you can find your own body making. Listen carefully. Your body might have a lot to say.

9. After a few moments of listening to your own body, gently open your eyes.

Follow-up: After practicing Layers of Sound, talk with your child about what she heard in each layer. Some children love to use a drawing activity after this practice to express the sounds that they heard, while others like to talk about them. Make sure that your child doesn't feel any pressure to identify the sounds—if she wants to share them with you she can just make the sounds out loud.

Challenges: The periods of silence in between each layer of sound are important parts of the activity, but they can be challenging for your child. If your child is finding this activity too long, or is struggling with the silence between layers, you can break up the practice by discussing or drawing what she heard after each layer, instead of all together at the end of the practice.

Daily Practice: Layers of Sound is a wonderful activity to practice before bedtime if your child struggles to fall asleep. Make sure you have introduced the activity during the day when your child is engaged; once it becomes comfortable and is no longer new, it is a very relaxing nighttime practice that can help reduce the impact of noise distractions keeping your child awake at night.

Walking Meditation

[handwritten note: Mountain pose → lean front & back → slow walk on mat → feeling in heels, toes, legs, hips, arms, body, neck & face → rhythm]

Practicing Walking Meditation is a grounding and steadying mindfulness activity that gives your child access to something that he can do anytime and anyplace when he needs to tune in to his own body and mind. It is a simple but supportive practice. The repetitive movement is soothing, and for many children the movement helps to quiet their minds. This is best done without shoes on.

1. Start off by getting grounded and connecting to your feet in mountain pose (see chapter 6). Stand in a tall and strong but also comfortable and relaxing position, with your feet hip-width apart.

2. Make sure your shoulders are relaxed, and take a few deep breaths.

3. Notice how your feet feel on the ground. Try moving your weight around a little to see how it feels. Lean forward and backward, then side to side. Then find the center—the place where you are balanced and most strong.

4. Begin taking a slow walk. If you are using a yoga mat, a good walking meditation path is to just walk from one end of the mat to the other and then turn around and walk back. Another great option is to do this outside in a safe place (grass is wonderful). If you aren't using a mat, you can walk a short path in any room and then turn around and walk back to where you started.

5. Start to notice how your feet feel as you walk. What is the sensation like in your heels? In your toes?

6. After a few moments, start to notice what walking feels like in the rest of your body. What happens in your legs and hips when you walk? What about your arms? Can you feel walking in your neck and your face?

7. Try to practice your walking long enough to notice the rhythm of your walk.

8. If your mind starts to wander while you are taking your walk, that's no problem. Just notice where it is wandering to and then gently bring it back to how your body is feeling during your walk.

9. When you are ready to finish your mindful walk, come back into mountain pose just like you started. Take a deep breath and send a thank-you thought to your feet.

Follow-up: Mindful walking is a great way for children to tune in to the sensations in their physical body. In fact, there are many other activities that your child does that can be similarly explored. Ask your child what it might feel like to mindfully take a ride on a swing, or to jump rope, or take a shower. Some children appreciate knowing that learning to tune in to their bodies while moving can help them become a better athlete.

Challenges: If this practice is a struggle for your child, you can invite him to walk in more playful ways. Ask, "What does it feel like to walk on your heels? On your toes? On the outside edges of your feet?" By changing the experience we increase engagement and ease of focus; however, as your child learns this activity, slowly reduce the amount of time spent walking playfully and reintroduce the simple mindful walk.

Daily Practice: As a daily practice, mindful walking keeps us grounded in our present experience and helps us stay connected to our bodies. It is best to give children (and yourself) a concrete and attainable goal. Try to get in the habit of making your first walk when you leave the house a mindful one. Setting an intention to walk mindfully to the car or school bus in the morning can have a powerful impact on the rest of your day.

Mindful Eating

Every day we think about food, prepare food, buy food, and eat food. But sometimes we are so busy that we forget to taste our food! Eating is an activity that we do several times a day, and it has the potential to bring us so much pleasure, but often both children and adults miss out on the sensations of eating because we are in a rush and distracted by other things. In this activity, we are going to explore all of the sensations of eating a clementine (one of the small, easy-to-peel kinds works best).

1. Pick up a clementine. Don't worry—you are going to get to eat it but not just yet.

2. First explore the clementine with your hands. Notice how heavy or light it is. Feel the texture of the skin and notice its temperature.

3. After you explore your clementine with your sense of touch, start to explore it with your sense of sight. Notice the color—is it even all the way around or does the color have variation in it? Notice if the skin is shiny or dull.

4. Now see if you can smell your clementine. First just hold it up to your nose. Then try scratching the skin and notice if it smells any different.

5. We now have two senses left to explore with: hearing and tasting. To use these senses we are going to have to peel our fruit. Start to peel your fruit slowly and carefully. Notice what the clementine feels like and looks like under the skin, and then as you are peeling hold it up to your ear. Does your clementine have anything to say?

6. Once your clementine is peeled, it is time to eat it! Go ahead and break off one section. Put it in your mouth but try not to chew at first.

7. Notice what the piece feels like in your mouth and what it tastes like on the outside. When you are ready to take a bite, do it slowly and notice everything—the taste, the feeling, your thoughts. Does the piece taste different on the inside and the outside? Can you feel it moving down your throat as you swallow?

8. When you are finished swallowing, start over with the next section of clementine, and notice if there is any difference between the two.

Follow-up: Be available to talk with your child after this practice and ask her about her experience. Throughout the day you can take advantage of moments to ask your child what she is experiencing through her senses. What is she smelling while dinner is cooking? What does she hear during a walk to school? What does she see during a car ride?

Challenges: If your child is a picky eater, it might help to let her choose the food the first time that she tries this practice. Other things that work well are raisins, carrots, and even ice cream cones, but you can really do this with any food. Don't be concerned if things get a little messy.

Daily Practice: Because we eat every day, making mindful eating a habit ensures that we are fully connecting to our present-moment experience of life a little bit each day. A useful practice is to try making the first bite of what you eat in the morning a mindful bite. If this works well for you, and starts to become a part of your life, you may want to try making the first bite of each meal a mindful bite.

Connecting with Your Self

When children (and adults) are overwhelmed it can be hard for them to stay connected to their emotional experience. Actions become automatic responses to input, and self-control becomes harder. The first step toward regulating your own behavior is recognizing your emotions, but when your attention is always being pulled outward, your own emotions often go unnoticed. Rapid changes in emotional state are common for many children. For children with ADHD, this tendency is even more pronounced, and because their impulse control is not very strong, rapid changes in behavior are also common. The first step toward self-regulation and meaningful decision making is learning to tune in to your emotions and feelings as they are arising.

The following activities all support the development of a healthy inner life for your child: both Checking In and Emotion Jar work to develop the habit of noticing the inner experience, Caring Feelings deepens and expands that inner awareness to others, and the I Am In Charge Mantra is a practical and easy exercise that creates a regular reminder to your child that she is the boss of her actions.

Checking In

Sometimes the most challenging part of connecting to how we are feeling is actually recognizing the feelings. Sometimes we are just so busy that we don't notice our feelings; sometimes feelings blur together and we only notice one of them (such as when we feel sad and angry at the same time but only notice the anger); and sometimes our feelings are just very confusing. Filling out the Checking-In Worksheet is a way to start becoming more aware of what you are experiencing in your body during different emotional states. Every person is different, and each person's body sends different messages to help him or her understand him- or herself better. Once you learn what your body's messages are, you can start to listen to those messages, reading your own body's clues to help you figure out what is happening with your emotions.

1. Before you introduce this worksheet, talk to your child about the idea of noticing emotions in our bodies. Provide examples such as clenching your fists when you are angry, or feeling butterflies in your belly when you are nervous. Ask your child if he has noticed any other ways that his feelings show up in his body.

2. Make two copies of the worksheet on the following pages, and during some quiet time introduce your child to the idea that if we can figure out what messages our bodies are sending us, we can understand ourselves better. Spend some time reading through the worksheet with your child; start with filling out just one emotion that he seems interested in.

3. Both you and your child should fill out worksheets during this activity. Discuss any similarities between the messages your bodies send, and any differences. Don't assume that your child will experience the same physical manifestations of emotion that you do.

4. Encourage your child to fill out the worksheet with words; also give him the option of drawing himself experiencing the emotion in the space available.

5. Don't worry about filling out the whole worksheet at once. It can take time to learn your body's messages. Keep the worksheet in an accessible place, and work on it during a week or two. If emotions come up that you want to explore that aren't on the worksheet, feel free to add them.

Follow-up: As your child learns more about his response to emotions, you can help support this development by compassionately pointing out situations when his body is giving him a clue that he doesn't notice. For example, you might say, "I can see that your eyebrows look scrunched." Being noticed in this way is very validating for your child. It tells him that you are tuned in to his experience and that you think his feelings are worth noticing.

Challenges: There may be some emotions that are harder than others to figure out, and there may be times when your child is too upset or too frustrated to notice what is happening. Take this activity slowly, and, especially in the beginning, don't ask your child to fill out the worksheet if he is having an intense emotional experience. See the A Guide to Compassionate Parenting in chapter 10 for guidance on communicating with your child during times of intense emotion.

Daily Practice: As you start to get into the habit of noticing your body's response to emotions, you will discover more nuances, and a richer emotional landscape will develop for you. Try printing a large version of this worksheet and hanging it on a wall where your child can access it. Throughout the day as he experiences different emotions, he may find that walking over to the worksheet and checking in can help him make sense of what he is feeling.

Checking-In Worksheet

Please photocopy the following pages or use them as an example to complete in your child's journal.

When I feel HAPPY what do I feel?   Drawing Space

My body: _____

_____

My breath: _____

_____

My belly: _____

_____

My face: _____

_____

When I feel FRUSTRATED what do I feel?

My body: _____

_____

My breath: _____

_____

My belly: _____

_____

My face: _____

_____

When I feel EXCITED what do I feel?   Drawing Space

My body: _____

_____

My breath: _____

_____

My belly: _____

_____

My face: _____

_____

When I feel ANGRY what do I feel?

My body: _____

_____

My breath: _____

_____

My belly: _____

_____

My face: _____

_____

When I feel SAD what do I feel?

My body: _____

_____

My breath: _____

_____

My belly: _____

_____

My face: _____

_____

When I feel NERVOUS what do I feel?

My body: _____

_____

My breath: _____

_____

My belly: _____

_____

My face: _____

Drawing Space

Emotion Jar

The Emotion Jar activity is a simple way to help remind your child to stay connected to her own feelings throughout the day, and to show her how feelings change over time. Creating opportunities for your child to check in with her feelings also shows her that you think her feelings are important and worth taking time to note. This validation strengthens your relationship and your capacity to help your child thrive. This activity was inspired in part by the work of Linda Lantieri. Her book and companion CD, *Building Emotional Intelligence*, is a great resource for more activities to help your child connect to her feelings.

1. Choose several clear containers to use as emotion jars. You can start with just a few, and then add to your collection as additional feelings become needed.

2. Gather some materials to create feeling labels for your jars. Large mailing labels work well, but you can also use paper and tape.

3. Think about some of the things that you feel during the day: happy, sad, tired, peaceful, excited, frustrated, angry, et cetera. Try starting with four or five emotions (some positive and some negative), and then adding to them the next time you work on this activity.

4. Make a label for each emotion. Write the name of the emotion and optionally draw a picture that goes with the feeling. Put one emotion label on each jar. Make one jar that reads "other" so that your child has an option if the emotions you've chosen don't fit at any particular time. Choose a place in your home where the jars can be displayed and easily accessed.

5. Now choose an object to represent yourself. (One good choice is a colored ping-pong ball—your child can even draw her face on it. If you have more than one child, you can use different objects or balls of different colors to represent each child. The adults in the home can participate as well.)

6. Close your eyes, take a full breath, and check in with your feelings. Choose the jar that best represents how you are feeling, and place your object in the jar. If there is no jar that represents how you feel, place your object in the "other" jar or make a new one.

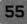

7. Now comes the tricky part. As you continue on with your day, try to pause every once in a while to check in. If you notice that the way you are feeling has changed, take the time to move your object to a different jar.

Follow-up: You child may have questions about this activity as she begins to pay more attention to her feelings. Make sure that you are available to talk; let her know that all emotions are important, even the ones that don't feel so great.

Challenges: The greatest challenge of the Emotion Jar activity is that sometimes it can be hard to know what you are feeling. Make sure your child knows that this is something you struggle with also—our feelings are complicated things, and it's possible to be having more than one feeling at the same exact time. If this is the case for your child, let her use more than one object in her jars.

Daily Practice: Emotion Jar is an activity that is best used on a daily basis. You want to reinforce the habit of tuning in to emotions and figuring out the names of less-familiar feelings. Make sure that you encourage your child to move her object to both positive and negative emotions. Remember, the goal is not to change your or your child's emotions or try to feel any particular way. The important part of this activity is to learn to notice all of your feelings, and to learn that you are still loved and accepted by your family when you have negative feelings.

Caring Feelings

The Caring Feelings activity is a child-friendly version of a Loving-Kindness or Metta practice, which is a type of meditation that can help your child develop compassion, contentment, and a feeling of well-being. In a traditional adult Loving-Kindness practice, kind thoughts would be sent to the self, to people close to you, to people you feel neutral about, and to people who you are angry or upset with. In our version, we are going to start with someone that your child loves very much, as this is the easiest way to access his kindness. We will end with the self, and, eventually, after this practice becomes familiar, you can try including someone challenging.

1. Begin by finding a comfortable seat; close your eyes.

2. Bring to mind someone that you love very much. This can be a family member or a friend. It can even be a pet. Imagine that person and begin to send caring feelings to that person. Notice how imagining this person makes your heart feel.

3. Now send some wishes to the person you've brought to mind. For instance, you can say, "May you be happy. May you be healthy. May you be peaceful. May you be filled with joy."

4. Next, send some kind thoughts to the people in your family—siblings, parents, aunts and uncles, and cousins. "May you be happy. May you be healthy. May you be peaceful. May you be filled with joy."

5. Now imagine sending loving kindness to children around the world—the ones who you know and the ones who you don't know. Imagine all of the children living around the world, the ones in your own neighborhood, and the ones who are living far away in other countries. Say to them, "May you be happy. May you be healthy. May you be peaceful. May you be filled with joy."

6. Finally, send loving kindness to yourself. Sometimes it can be challenging to send kind wishes and caring feelings to yourself, but, if you learn how, you will

always be able to give yourself a boost of love when you need it. Imagine yourself sitting in a quiet place where you feel comfortable and safe. Now say to yourself three times, "May I be happy. May I be healthy. May I be peaceful. May I be filled with joy."

7. Sit quietly for a moment or two, then open your eyes. (When practicing with your child, you can ring the singing bowl, to let him know that it's time to open his eyes.)

Follow-up: Ask your child how he felt about sending out the caring feelings, especially how it felt sending them to himself. You might talk about times when he sent unkind feelings to others or to himself, and how that felt. Ask him if there is anyone else he would like to send caring feelings to before you finish up for the day.

Challenges: Once this activity becomes familiar, try including a person that your child has a hard time with in his kind thoughts. Be sure to avoid anyone who your child finds frightening or is extremely angry at. Instead, try using language like "someone who annoys you" or "someone who has been bugging you lately."

Daily Practice: Caring Feelings is a wonderful practice to bring into your daily life, as an antidote to the negative thoughts we all have about ourselves from time to time. Encourage your child to send himself kind and caring thoughts throughout the day, especially if he is feeling a little bit down. As the practice gets familiar, you can both experiment with sending kind thoughts to someone after an argument or disagreement (especially if you have an argument with each other!). Explain to your child that sending kind thoughts to someone else is a way to help himself feel better, even if he is still upset with the other person.

I Am In Charge Mantra

This children's meditation is a variation on a traditional *kundalini* yoga meditation. It is an active meditation that reinforces your child's personal power and capacity for self-determination. It is accessible and engaging for children who have trouble keeping their bodies still, and for many children this becomes one of their most relied-upon tools in everyday life.

1. This meditation combines vocalization with movement of your fingers. You will connect each of your fingers to your thumb on both hands at once, while reciting the mantra "I am in charge."

2. Say one word at a time as you connect your fingers. Press your thumb and first finger together saying "I," your thumb and middle finger together saying "am," your thumb and ring finger together saying "in," and your thumb and pinkie together saying "charge."

3. Put enough pressure on your fingers to really feel the connection they are making. Once you get into the rhythm of the practice, close your eyes and keep going, repeating the movement and the mantra for as long as you choose, starting out with just a few moments and then working up to several minutes.

4. Begin slowly, using both hands simultaneously, and, as you feel more comfortable, go a bit faster. You can start saying "I am in charge" loudly and then lower your voice with each round until it becomes a whisper, ultimately repeating it silently to yourself for a few rounds.

5. The mantra "I am in charge" is a very useful one, but you can also try this meditation with any four-word (or four-syllable) mantra or saying. Feel free to experiment and be creative. Some examples are "I am so strong" or "I will be kind." Your child may enjoy creating her own mantra, but once she has chosen a mantra (after trying a few), encourage her to stick with and practice that one specific mantra. Through repetition it will become a part of how she thinks about herself and serve as a touchstone for gathering strength in challenging situations.

Follow-up: The mantra "I am in charge" raises the question of what you are in charge of. Take the time to talk with your child about the things in life that we all control for ourselves. Children often feel like they have very little control and self-determination in their lives. Help your child explore where she has choices and ways that she has control over her experiences, actions, and reactions.

Challenges: Younger children or those with fine-motor challenges may struggle with the coordination to connect their fingers, especially with their eyes closed. Encourage them to practice the movement first, and even to watch their fingers if they need to, and then add the vocalization as the movement becomes comfortable.

Daily Practice: This activity gains potency with repetition. Encourage your child to practice it for just a couple of moments each day, and then to use it anytime she feels like she needs some extra personal power. This can even be done in the classroom when she feels particularly restless, if she moves her fingers silently. For many children this small movement can help them stay calm and connected during the school day.

Taking a Step-by-Step Approach

Each of these activities has value both in what happens during the activity and what happens to the habits of the mind when the activity becomes part of your way of living. Connecting to the environment and connecting to the self need to become habits for your child, routine practices that, over time, become a normal part of how he operates in the world. For yoga and mindfulness practice to have the greatest impact on your child's everyday life, make them a part of the everyday life of your family.

When you first begin to introduce these Connect activities to your child, think of them as a chance to explore. Encourage your child to ask questions, and share your own feelings and thoughts about the practices. Reinforce the idea that there is no one right way to do these activities, and keep the mood light and playful. The activities that your child is most responsive to and interested in should be the ones that you focus on including in daily practice. As the activities are repeated you can start practicing them with more intention—working on keeping your body still, keeping your eyes closed, or increasing the length of the practice.

While you may have purchased this book with one family member in mind, all of the activities will benefit anyone. I encourage you to share the practices with your whole family and view them as a path toward developing a more integrated and fulfilling way of life. Embracing the program as a family will change the way your child experiences it. Instead of being singled out as having a problem that needs to be fixed, your child will be part of a collaborative effort to live a healthy and happy life.

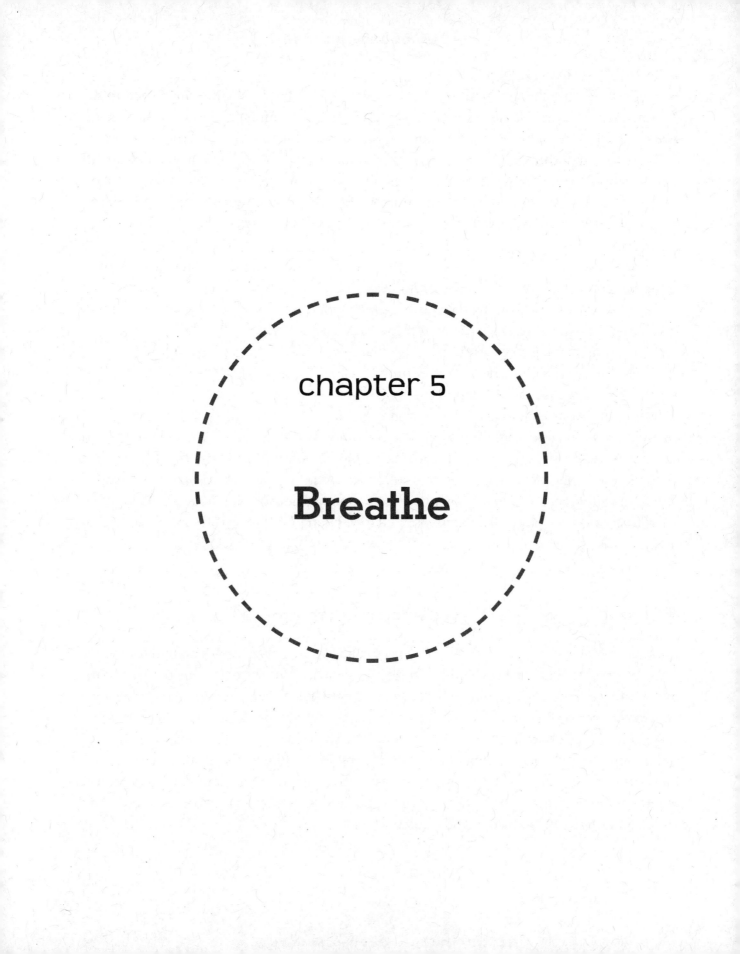

chapter 5

Breathe

Let's begin this chapter by trying a short experiment. Find a comfortable place to sit where you won't be disturbed or distracted for a few minutes. Set up an alarm to sound in one minute, and for that minute close your eyes and breathe in and out through your mouth. Notice any feelings that come up for you either in your body or in your emotional state. When the alarm goes off, open your eyes, remember how you felt, and set the alarm again. Now, for one minute, breathe in and out through your nose. Notice how this makes you feel, and note any differences between these two experiences.

How did you feel? Did you notice a big difference? When I do this experiment with a group of people, I generally get responses like:

"I felt so uncomfortable breathing through my mouth."

"When I breathed through my mouth I wanted to open my eyes."

"Breathing through my mouth felt hard, like I couldn't do it right."

"Breathing through my nose felt soothing."

"I felt much calmer breathing through my nose."

What was your experience? Would you ever have imagined that just one minute of changing your breath would make such a tremendous difference in your physical and emotional well-being? In yoga, the breath is considered our most powerful tool for directly impacting our energetic and emotional state. In Sanskrit, the traditional language of yoga, the word for "breath" is "*prana*," which is the same as the word for "energy." When we want to change our physical or emotional energy, changing the way we are breathing is the most effective way to do it.

Why Does Your Breath Matter?

In order to make sense of why our breath has such a big impact on us, it's helpful to understand a little bit about the involuntary actions of our nervous systems. Our bodies are in many ways governed by two different masters: *the sympathetic nervous system* and the *parasympathetic nervous system*. The parasympathetic system regulates our normal metabolic functions—things like digestion, healing, and growth. When our parasympathetic system is dominant, our bodies can function optimally, and for children this means that they can grow and develop in a healthy way. When our parasympathetic system is in charge, we breathe in and out through our noses. This is the healthiest way for our bodies to breathe, as the air coming in is warmed and filtered.

The sympathetic nervous system is what we generally think of as our fight, flight, or freeze mode. It's the part of us that takes control when we feel threatened or fearful (it's one of the great tools of the Protective Brain, which we discuss in chapter 1). When the sympathetic nervous system is in charge, all of our normal metabolic functions are put on hold, we experience a flood of adrenaline into our bodies, and our energy is diverted to physical strength and increased alertness so that we can run or fight. When the sympathetic nervous system is activated, we breathe in and out through our mouths in order to take in the most oxygen as quickly as possible.

In an ideal world, our sympathetic nervous system would only be activated when there was a genuine threat to our safety. Most of the time, we would be using our energy to stay healthy, digest our food, process toxins from our body, and grow. The problem is that for many people, both adults and children, the sympathetic nervous system gets stuck in the on position even when there is no genuine threat. This can happen for many different reasons. Too much sensory stimulation (including bright lights and loud noises, which are very common in urban environments), chronic stress, previous trauma, and persistent anxiety can all contribute to a situation whereby our bodies feel that they need to be on high alert on a regular basis.

When that happens, we end up with all sorts of problems, from stomachaches to compromised immune function and, in extreme cases, even delayed growth. When our sympathetic nervous system is overactivated, it also makes it very challenging to stay focused. Usually, when we need to focus on something, our mind helps by adjusting to and filtering out irrelevant stimuli, but when our sympathetic nervous system is in charge, every noise, sight, and smell represents a potential danger that has to be evaluated. Our decision making is also impacted, as we are in a state of high reactivity, where the body responds to input and impulses quickly and defensively.

With this understanding of the sympathetic and parasympathetic nervous systems, we can make more sense of why our breath has such a strong effect on how we feel. When the parasympathetic nervous system is in control, we breathe through our nose. When the sympathetic nervous system is in control, we breathe through our mouth. What is remarkable is that the reverse is also true. When you breathe through your mouth, you send a signal to your body that it needs to be ready for something, and the sympathetic nervous system starts to take control. When you breathe through your nose, you are telling your body that everything is okay. The parasympathetic system can take over. You can heal, digest, learn, and grow.

What this means is that if breathing through your nose becomes a habit, and you deliberately breathe through your nose in times of challenge, you can actually begin to change the response of your nervous system and override your body's fight-flight-or-freeze response. Of course, breathing through your nose when your body is reacting to stress, anxiety, or fear is not always easy. Learning to notice your breathing, and then make the effort to change it, is a skill that can be practiced. By teaching our children that they are the masters of their breath, we can help them shift their way of interacting with their own emotions and with the world around them.

Bringing Energy Up and Down

Your breath also has a powerful ability to help you manage your energy level. The quality of your breath—the pacing, the depth, the ratio of your inhale to exhale—can be used intentionally and effectively to help both you and your child get energized or calm down. The practices in this section will give you options for both, but the healthiest default state of breath for your child is to breathe slowly through his nose on both the inhale and the exhale. As he practices these activities, your child will naturally begin to become more aware of how he is breathing during the day. Encourage him to notice when he starts breathing through his mouth, and then have him practice switching to nose breathing.

The Practices

The activities described in the following pages are meant to increase both breath awareness and breath control. They are all based on a foundation of full breathing through the nose. If your child tends to breathe through her mouth often, it might be useful to spend the first session or two of breathwork just focusing on switching to nose-based breathing.

You can do this in a very simple way by sitting together in a quiet place and deliberately breathing in and out through the nose with your child. If she is used to breathing through her mouth, this might feel strange at first. Breathing through your nose slows down your breath, and kids who are generally moving at a very fast pace might struggle with this feeling of slowness. Don't worry about your child mastering nose-based breathing before starting the activities that follow. Just expose her to the idea a few times, then give the activities a try.

Many kids are familiar with the expression "take a deep breath." This is something they have likely heard from you or from other adults in their lives at times when they were upset, angry, frustrated, or otherwise struggling to control their emotions. Sometimes, taking a deep breath leads kids to overemphasize their inhalation, filling up with air in an uncomfortable way that contributes to, rather than reduces, anxiety. For both of these reasons, I prefer to avoid telling children to take a deep breath. Instead, focus on the idea of taking a full, comfortable breath in, and then exhaling all of your air out completely.

A note about asthma: Many children with asthma find breathwork to be empowering. For the first time, they feel some control over something that is often scary, and this can help reduce some of the anxiety that comes with their asthma. These practices are gentle, but if you are nervous about your child's asthma, be sure to talk with your doctor about your concerns, and seek his or her advice on the activities in this section. Remember the importance of our discussion in chapter 3—children should not be pressured to do anything that feels uncomfortable for them in any way. If your child begins to feel anxious, uncomfortable, or nervous during breathwork activities, stop right away and talk with her about what she felt. Try reducing the length of time you are practicing, or choose to focus just on a simple inhale and exhale through the nose. Let your child decide if and when she is ready to try the activity again.

Balloon Breath

Balloon Breath is a simple practice that incorporates a repetitive movement of the body with the breath pattern. This is very supportive for children who initially struggle with controlling their breath. It also serves to open the chest and gently stretch the back of the shoulders, releasing some of the physical tension that might be contributing to shallow breathing.

1. Begin this practice by sitting somewhere comfortable with your child, either on the floor or in a chair, with your back straight and tall. Place your hands on your knees and start to breathe in and out through your nose.

2. Now imagine that your body is a balloon, and with each breath in you are filling yourself completely with air. As you breathe in, arch your back, let your chest and belly soften and move forward, and look up. This is a modified form of cat pose (see chapter 6).

3. As you breathe out, pull your belly button in, round your back, and look down toward your belly. This is a modified form of cow pose (see chapter 6).

4. Repeat this movement and breath pattern several times, breathing in to fill up your body and breathing out to deflate it.

5. On your next inhale, repeat the opening of your chest but this time bring your arms up and over your head as well. Make your body very big and full. (See illustration 1.)

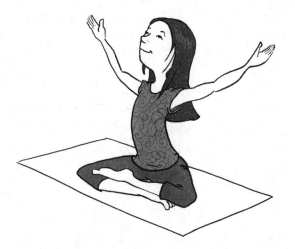

Illustration 1: Balloon breath—on the inhale, with arms extended

6. As you breathe out, bring your arms back down. As you round your back and pull in your belly, wrap your arms around yourself in a hug. (See illustration 2.)

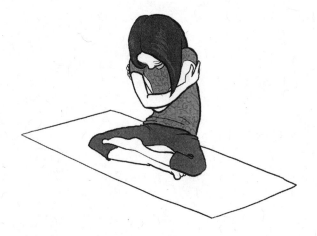

Illustration 2: Balloon breath—on the exhale

7. Continue for a few rounds, breathing in to fill yourself up and get very big, and breathing out to make yourself as small as you can be.

Follow-up: The pattern of movement described here is just one possible way to practice this breath. If your child enjoys this combination of breathing and movement, go ahead and explore other ways to move. The important thing is that the body is opening and expanding when you breathe in, and getting smaller as you breathe out.

Challenges: If your child is having a particularly high-energy day, there could be a temptation here to move the body very quickly and let the breath follow in a counterproductive way. Make sure that you set the pace of the breath first, before you start moving the body, and encourage your child to let the movement take the entire length of the breath to complete.

Daily Practice: Balloon Breath is a great way to start your day. It's a way to take the natural stretching and yawning that often happens in the morning and make it more productive and intentional. Suggest to your child that he try a few moments of Balloon Breath first thing in the morning, right in his bed, to help wake up his breath and his body.

Heart and Belly Breath

This practice is a beautiful way to teach children a basic *samavritti* breath, which is an even and steady inhalation and exhalation. It is a very comforting activity that children can integrate easily into their daily life. The combination of slow, steady breathing with the simple connection of the hands to the body almost immediately calm the nervous system. Many children (and adults) find this to be one of their favorite practices.

1. You can do this activity sitting or lying down. If you're going to sit, find a comfortable seat where you won't need to shift around, and sit as tall as you can. If you decide to lie down, do it where you won't be disturbed and where you feel comfortable and safe.

2. Place one hand on your belly and one hand over your heart (in the center of your chest).

3. Before you start doing anything special with your breath, take a moment to notice how your breath is moving into and out of your body. Notice where you can most feel your breath in your body (nose, chest, belly, back, etc.). Observe if your breath feels relaxed or tight.

4. Now start to breathe a little bit more mindfully. Breathe in and out through your nose, and as you breathe in, let your belly get softer and bigger, filling with air. As you breathe out, pull your belly button in, pushing all of the air out.

5. Breathe in this pattern for a few moments, focusing on moving your breath into and out of your belly. It can be very helpful to establish the rhythm of your child's breath by counting aloud for her, *Inhale one, two; exhale one, two.* Make sure that the counting matches a full comfortable breath for your child—don't try to make her breath go in or out for longer than feels good.

6. After a few rounds, it's time to start breathing into the heart also. The next time you breathe in, fill your belly with air. Then breathe in a little bit more and fill the space behind your heart with air. When it's time to exhale, let your breath go from behind your heart, then squeeze the rest out of your belly.

7. Counting is even more helpful here. Consider counting out loud as your child practices: *Into your belly one, two, into your heart three, four; out of your heart one, two, out of your belly three, four.*

Follow-up: Heart and Belly Breath has a strong energetic effect on most people. Try to encourage your child to sit quietly for a moment or two after finishing this practice, as a way to notice any feelings she is having and to transition gently to whatever is coming next.

Challenges: If your child is having a hard time with the coordination of this practice (or if you think she might), feel free to start by just breathing into and out of the belly, without bringing the breath into and out of the heart. You can add the heart component at any time, even if it is weeks or months after learning the initial activity. If you decide to do this, I still recommend that you have the hands placed over both the belly and the heart, as the physical contact is very soothing even without the addition of the heart breath.

Daily Practice: Heart and Belly Breath is an easy and effective way to tune in and help calm yourself down at any point during the day. Let your child know that if she feels overwhelmed, frustrated, or like things just aren't feeling right, Heart and Belly Breath can often help. This is also a great practice to use as an opening ritual for your regular yoga sessions together. (See chapter 3 for more on opening rituals.)

Langhana and Brahmana Breath

This activity features two different, simple ways to breathe in order to change your energy level. *Langhana* breath brings your energy down; it's quieting and calming and encourages an inward focus. *Brahmana* breath revitalizes you; it is stimulating and energizing with a quality of alertness.

Langhana Breath

In this practice there is a greater awareness and attention placed on the exhale, which should be longer than the inhale.

1. Start in a seated position, with your eyes closed, and breathe through your nose for a few breaths.

2. Begin to silently count your breathing pattern, for example, *Inhale one, two; exhale one, two...* (you may want to count out loud for your child). Make sure that the count isn't too long and that your child can comfortably inhale and exhale for the counted length of the breath.

3. Once you are breathing at a steady pace for a few rounds, start to make your exhale longer than your inhale. You can start by counting, *Inhale one, two; exhale one, two, three.* If this feels okay, try *Inhale one, two; exhale one, two, three, four....*

4. Continue this pattern for as long as you feel comfortable. When you're ready to finish, come back to an even breath for a round or two, and then gently open your eyes.

Brahmana Breath

In this practice there is a greater awareness and attention placed on the inhale, which should be longer than the exhale.

1. Start in a seated position, with your eyes closed, and breathe through your nose for a few breaths.

2. Begin to silently count your breathing pattern, for example, *Inhale one, two; exhale one, two...* (you may want to count out loud for your child). Make sure that the count isn't too long and that your child can comfortably inhale and exhale for the counted length of the breath.

3. Once you are breathing at a steady pace for a few rounds, start to make your inhale longer than your exhale. You can start by counting, *Inhale one, two, three; exhale one, two.* If this feels okay, try *Inhale one, two, three, four; exhale one, two....*

4. Make sure that you are getting all of your air out on the exhale. This might mean that you need to exhale more strongly than usual.

5. Continue this pattern for as long as you feel comfortable. When you're ready to finish, come back to an even breath for a round or two, and then gently open your eyes.

Follow-up: Encourage your child to pay close attention to how these two ways of breathing make him feel. When you are just starting to practice *langhana* and *brahmana* breathing, it can be useful to do them one after the other to help explore the different feelings that they generate, but you can also just practice one of them based on what you think your child needs at the time.

Challenges: Some children struggle with *brahmana* breath, as the inhale can get too long, making it a little bit uncomfortable. Work with your child to find an inhale length that feels full but that doesn't cause him any anxiety. Remind your child that if something doesn't feel right he can always tell you, and that you'll be okay with working on something else.

Daily Practice: These breathing patterns are extremely useful in daily life. Once your child becomes comfortable with them, remind him that he always has a way to control his energy level. Anytime he needs to calm his energy down, he can try practicing *langhana* breath, and if he needs to wake himself up he can practice *brahmana* breath.

Alternate-Nostril Breathing

Alternate-Nostril Breathing helps neutralize your child's energy and emotions. The goal of this practice is not necessarily to calm down, but to bring balance and a sense of stability to the moment. Give your child some time to get used to this because it both looks and feels very strange.

1. Find a comfortable seat, and sit up tall.

2. Before you start this activity, take a few slow, full belly breaths through your nose.

3. Tell your child that the part that comes next is going to look really silly. We are going to use our fingers to close off our nostrils one at a time and alternate breathing through each of them.

4. Bring your right hand up to your nose and demonstrate the two positions that your child can choose from. In the first, the index finger and middle finger are curled into the palm, and the thumb and ring fingers are resting on either nostril. In the second, the index and ring fingers are resting above the bridge of the nose.

5. Give her a minute to choose a hand position and get the giggles out.

6. Now close off your left nostril with your ring finger. Breathe in through your open right nostril. (See illustration 3.)

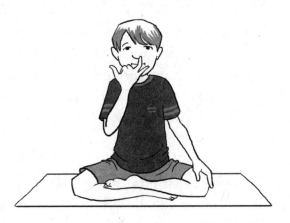

Illustration 3: Alternate-nostril breathing

7. Then close your right nostril with your thumb, and open your left nostril to breathe out.

8. Breathe in through your open left nostril.

9. Close your left nostril, open your right, and breathe out through your right.

10. Then breathe in through your right, close it, and breathe out through your left.

11. Make sure that you start this slowly and let your child get used to what she is doing. Guide her through one step at a time with plenty of pauses to integrate the instructions.

12. Once she starts getting the hang of it, continue to give guidance but use fewer words. Establish a rhythm to the breathing by repeating, *In right, out left, in left, out right,* and so on.

13. Keep going in this pattern for a few minutes.

14. As you finish the exercise, release your hand and take a few slow breaths in and out of both nostrils.

Follow-up: It might take a few tries for this to start feeling like it makes sense, but once your child gets the hang of it, take a few minutes after she is finished to ask her to check in with her body and emotions, and notice any feelings or sensations.

Challenges: If the work of coordinating the hand movements seems distracting, make sure you spend a little bit of time playing with the hand movements alone, independent of the breath. When your child feels comfortable with the hand movements, then introduce the breath and put the two together.

Daily Practice: Alternate-Nostril Breathing can be used anytime your child feels like she needs to hit a reset button. It works equally well in situations where she wants to calm herself down or give herself a little more energy. Because it is energetically balancing, it's a great practice to try when things don't feel quite right, but you aren't sure exactly what you need to feel balanced.

Back-to-Back Breathing

Back-to-Back Breathing is a partner activity that you and your child can practice together, or that you can introduce to siblings or friends. It is a favorite activity of many children and adults, as it feels supportive, loving, and nurturing. It is a way to soothe both you and your child, as well as a way to deepen your connection with each other.

1. Start by sitting back to back on the floor, with your legs crossed in front of you. Try to sit close together and very straight, so that as much of your back as possible is touching your child's back. Go ahead and lean into each other a little.

2. Close your eyes and start to breathe in and out through your nose. With each breath, fill your whole body up with air. (See illustration 4.)

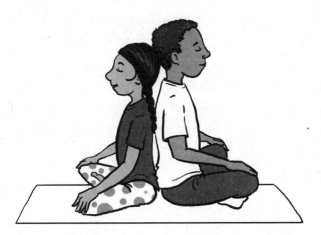

Illustration 4: Back-to-back breathing

3. After a few moments start to see if you can feel your partner's breath moving in his body. Can you feel his back or shoulders moving just a little? Can you hear his breath at all?

4. Without talking, try to begin matching your breath to your partner's breath, and begin breathing in and out together.

5. Stay here for a few minutes, lightly leaning on each other and breathing together.

6. You can continue this for as long as it feels good for both of you. When you are ready to get up, do so slowly and carefully, being gentle with your partner.

Follow-up: Avoid having a lot of conversation around this activity with your child. The experience itself is the important thing, and sometimes talking about the sense of connection and support can make your child feel silly or uncomfortable. Unless he brings up a conversation around this practice, just let the experience stand on its own.

Challenges: In order to feel the full impact of this practice, it's important for the partners to stay connected to each other, which can be challenging for a child who is struggling to stay still. If this is happening, try to experiment with things that can help create a sense of grounding for your child. For example, you can do this practice with your hands on your heart and belly. You can also try draping a blanket around the two of you. Choose the time of day for this practice carefully, when you know that your child will be more likely to feel calm and be capable of a few moments of stillness.

Daily Practice: Back-to-Back Breathing is not something that I generally recommend trying to incorporate into your child's everyday routine, but it is very nourishing to practice it on a regular basis (maybe four or five times per month) depending on how much you are both enjoying it.

Using Your Breath in Challenging Situations

As you and your child practice the breathing activities in this chapter, you are both likely to become more aware of your breath in ordinary circumstances. This is a wonderful gift, as breath awareness will give you a tremendous amount of insight into your energetic and emotional state. Revisit the Checking-In Worksheet that your child created during the Connect practices to remind him of how he can use his breath to give him clues about his emotions. As greater breath awareness allows him to notice more, continue to add to the worksheet.

Remind your child that his breath is his to control. He has the power to turn his energy up or down, to help himself relax, or even to make himself more upset. Encourage him to notice his breath throughout the day and make decisions about whether he wants to change it. Remember that just because this is all possible doesn't mean it is easy! It takes a tremendous amount of self-awareness and self-control to use your breath mindfully in difficult situations. Your child is just starting to learn these skills, and you are helping him practice. Don't expect immediate mastery, and don't let your enthusiasm for these practices diminish how seriously you take your child's emotions. Make sure that you honor his feelings and that he always knows that you're on his side.

Remember that you can use all of these tools as a parent also. When you are frustrated, angry, or even afraid, try to notice your breath and make a decision about whether to change it. During particularly challenging moments, pause and let your child know that you are working with your breath to calm yourself down. Practice these activities with your child, and practice them on your own. Model the skillful use of your breath and it will influence your entire family.

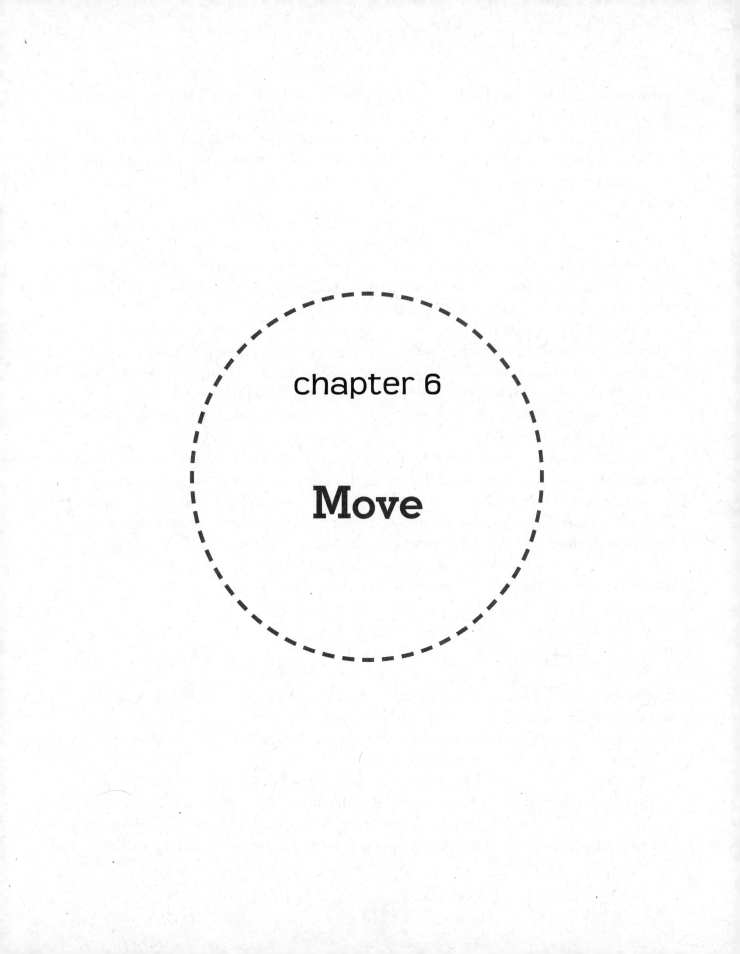

chapter 6

Move

For many children, movement is their natural state of being. Kids fidget, run around, and bounce in their seats, and sometimes it seems like the last thing we would want is to get them moving more. When we ask our kids to focus or to pay attention, one of the things we often want is for them to stop moving. Yet movement in the body can have a tremendously positive impact on a child's emotional well-being and on her capacity to focus.

While parents and teachers may interpret a child's stillness as attentiveness, in our own lives we find ourselves pacing when we are trying to solve a problem, shifting in our seats while we listen to a lecture or watch a play, and going for a run when we feel overwhelmed. We intuitively know that by moving our bodies we are affecting our minds, and research confirms this is true for both children and adults.

Movement has a positive impact on anxiety, stress, and general mental health. Yoga programs have been shown to increase executive function in children, including improving focus and reducing impulsivity (Diamond and Lee 2011). "The flow of energy and information from the body up into our brain stem, into our limbic region, and then up into the cortex, changes our bodily states, our emotional states, and our thoughts" (Siegel and Bryson 2011, 61).

The yoga poses discussed in this chapter will teach your child to use her body in an intentional way, so that movement helps generate and maintain a state of engaged alertness. Frenetic and hyperactive energy is reduced, yet she will still feel vibrant and strong. The goal of these Move activities is to validate your child's inclination to be active, while giving her the tools to make choices about it. The objective is not to send the message to your child that she just "needs to calm down" but rather that she can be mindful of her actions and find an enjoyable balance of energy and stillness.

The Practices

The following Move activities are presented in three categories—grounding, strength, and balance. While you can practice one activity at a time, choosing one activity from each category to practice in sequence will give a more well-rounded experience and will leave your child feeling energetically balanced.

Remember when you start these activities with your child that all movement in yoga is about exploration. At some point, your child is likely to ask you if she is doing the pose "right." This can be a tricky question to answer, because the real impact of the movement comes not from the shape of the pose but from the child's intention, effort, and attitude.

When your child asks if she is doing a pose right, try to answer with some version of "You can't tell from the outside if a yoga pose is right." Some children resist this type of answer because they are very achievement oriented; they want some way to measure their ability and the external validation of getting it "right." Talk about all of the ways your child can figure out for herself if she is having a good yoga experience. Ask some questions such as: "How do your arms feel? Is your breath steady? Do you feel strong?" Point out that she can decide for herself if she is doing the pose right, by making sure that nothing hurts, that her breath is steady, and that she is focusing on what she is doing at the moment.

Warming Up: Cat, Cow, and Twist Poses

At the beginning of any Move practice, consider taking a few minutes to gently warm up your body with the following simple cat and cow stretches, plus a twist, particularly if you are planning on doing some of the more challenging poses.

1. Start on your hands and knees in the middle of your mat. Make sure that your hands are directly under your shoulders and that your knees are directly under your hips.

2. Spread out your fingers.

3. Take a full breath in and arch your back, pulling your shoulders down and looking up toward the ceiling. This is cow pose. (See illustration 5.)

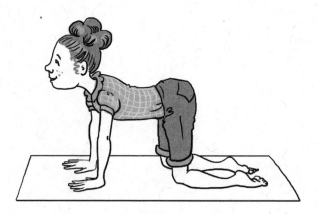

Illustration 5: Cow pose

4. As you breathe out, round your back, spreading your shoulder blades apart and looking toward your belly. This is cat pose. (See illustration 6.)

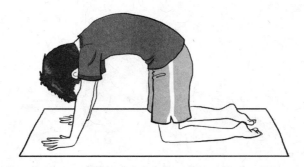

Illustration 6: Cat pose

5. Repeat this three to five times, moving slowly and breathing fully with each movement.

6. After three to five rounds of cat and cow poses, bring your back to neutral (nice and flat).

7. Slide your right arm underneath your left shoulder, twisting to the left and bringing your shoulder and ear to your mat. (See illustration 7.) Rest here for three breaths and then come back to the middle slowly. Twist to the other side for three breaths.

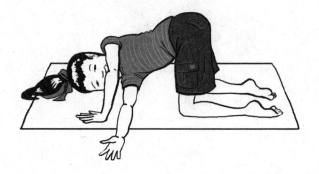

Illustration 7: A gentle twist following cat and cow poses

8. Come back to the middle, and rest for a moment or two in child's pose (see next pose) before moving on to the rest of your practice.

A Place to Rest: Child's Pose

While you and your child are practicing the activities that follow, remember that it is always up to you to take care of yourself and rest when you need to (or even when you just want to). Child's pose is a safe, nurturing way to give your body a break at any point in your yoga practice.

1. Come onto your hands and knees in the middle of your mat.

2. Sit your hips back onto your heels, and fold forward to lay your chest over your thighs.

3. You can keep your knees together here, or if it feels more comfortable you can open your knees wider and let your chest come down between them. The idea is to let your body rest, so experiment with what feels most relaxing for you.

4. If you can reach it comfortably, let your forehead rest on the mat. If it doesn't reach the ground, you can rest your forehead on a folded blanket or a block.

5. Either stretch your arms out in front of you, or pull them back to rest alongside your body. Choose whichever variation is more comfortable for you. (See illustration 8.)

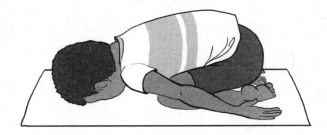

Illustration 8: Child's pose

6. Stay here as long as you want, taking slow, full breaths and giving yourself a rest.

Grounding: Mountain Pose

Mountain pose is a fundamental starting point for all standing poses in the yoga practice. It is an easy way to check in with your body at any point during the day. It's also a good alternative to sitting for Breathe and Focus activities, if you don't feel like sitting down during your practice.

1. Start by standing with your feet either hip-width apart or close together with your big toes touching. Either way, your feet should be parallel to each other. To check this, look at the outside edges of your feet.

2. Stand up tall and think about making your whole body strong and steady but relaxed, starting with your feet.

3. Wiggle your toes, then spread them out and place them back down. Imagine your feet getting very heavy and sinking into the support of the ground.

4. Check to make sure that your knees aren't locked. Pull your belly in and move your shoulders back. Let your arms relax by your sides, and turn them so that your palms are facing forward.

5. Hold your head tall and relax your face.

6. Take a full breath in and grow a little taller. Breathe out and get a little more relaxed.

Follow-up: Check in with your child. Ask her how her body feels in mountain pose. Make sure she knows that it is perfectly normal to find standing still a tremendous challenge. If your child seems to get the wiggles after mountain pose, try moving beforehand instead, letting her shake out each part of her body, and then begin her practice.

Challenges: For many people, both children and adults, poses that require stillness are the hardest ones of all. If your child is fidgeting or uncomfortable practicing mountain pose, try offering her a chant or a saying that she can repeat either silently or out loud during the practice. You can create your own saying with your child, but something connected to the pose, such as "I am as strong as a mountain. I am steady through wind and rain," would work well.

Daily Practice: Mountain pose can be incorporated into daily life during all of the moments when your child has to stand still but may be feeling impatient, such as while waiting in line. It is also a great way to start the day. Encourage your child to take a few breaths in mountain pose the first time her feet hit the floor in the morning.

Grounding: Malasana

Malasana, sometimes called "garland pose" or "frog pose," is a deep squat that brings your body very close to the ground. It stretches open your hips, strengthens your legs and your core muscles, and opens your chest. This is a pose that is often easier for children than for their parents!

1. Begin by standing in mountain pose (see previous pose). Then separate your feet to about the width of your shoulders (or a little farther if it's comfortable). Pointing your toes out a tiny bit will help you get into this pose.

2. Now reach your arms straight out in front of you, and slowly begin to bend your knees and lower your hips. Come all the way down into a squatting position, with your hips very low but not quite touching the ground.

3. Bring your hands together at the center of your chest, and put your elbows on the inside of your knees. Gently push your hands together, and push your knees a little farther apart. Lift your chest so you are sitting tall. (See illustration 9.)

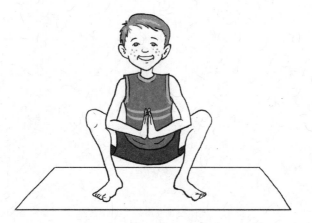

Illustration 9: Malasana

4. When you first try this pose, hold it for two or three slow, steady breaths. As you become stronger and more flexible, you can stay here for as many as six to eight breaths.

Follow-up: After practicing *malasana*, it might feel good to stand up and gently fold forward, just letting your body dangle softly, even swaying from side to side or front to back (see rag doll pose in chapter 11). When you're ready, roll up to standing.

Challenges: *Malasana* can be tough if you don't have a lot of natural flexibility in your hips. If your heels don't comfortably come to rest on the floor in this pose, you can help yourself by rolling or folding a section of your yoga mat or a blanket to a thickness of a few inches and placing it under your heels.

Daily Practice: Let your child know that in many indigenous cultures around the world, squatting is the way people spend much of their day. Instead of sitting in chairs, they might squat to cook, eat, talk, or play games. Invite your child to experiment with how it would feel to live without chairs and couches. Any activity that is usually done seated can be done in *malasana* instead, with a lot of benefits for your body.

Grounding: Seated Forward Bends

Seated forward bends are important poses that help bring a calming energy to your body. When the world feels overwhelming, a seated forward bend can be a soothing way to settle both your body and your mind. The basic principles of seated forward bends are the same for each variation, but as you change the position of your legs, different muscles are stretched.

Straight-Leg Forward Bend

1. Sit on your mat with both legs stretched straight out in front of you. Sit up very straight and tall. It's important that you aren't leaning back at all and that your body is lifting straight up over your hips.

2. Look down at your toes and gently flex your feet (bring your toes toward your body).

3. Check to make sure that your knees aren't locked, and if they are, bend them a tiny bit.

4. Now bring your hands over your heart (in the center of your chest), and imagine that a string tied right at that spot is pulling you straight forward. Move your chest forward and start to reach your hands and arms forward as well. This part is very important—your body should move forward, not down toward your legs (at least not yet). Try to keep your spine nice and long, and reach out as far as you can with your hands and your heart. Keep flexing your feet toward your body. (See illustration 10.)

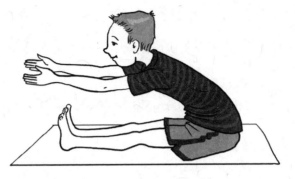

Illustration 10: Seated forward bend—reaching forward to achieve length in the spine

5. Once you've gotten as long as possible, relax and lower your body down toward your legs. You can stay here for as long as it feels good, but try to stay a little longer each time you practice. (See illustration 11.)

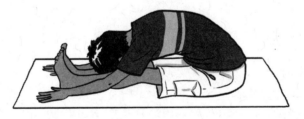

Illustration 11: Seated forward bend—lowering the torso to relax

6. When you are finished, a simple backbend will feel great to neutralize your spine. Start from the same seated position, then bend your knees and put your feet on the ground. Then bring your hands back behind you (under your shoulders) with your fingers facing your hips. Gently push into your hands and feet, and lift your hips so that they are about as high as your knees. This is known as tabletop pose. Hold for a few breaths, then return to sitting.

Bound-Ankle Pose

1. Sit on your mat with the soles of your feet together and your knees open.

2. Don't try to push your knees down toward the ground, just relax them and let gravity do the work. This is also known as butterfly pose.

3. Now follow steps 4 to 6 for the straight-leg forward bend pose. (See illustration 12.)

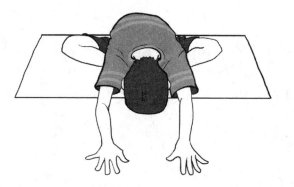

Illustration 12: Bound-ankle pose

Head-to-Knee Pose

1. Sit down and extend one leg straight out in front of you.

2. Bend the other knee, and place the sole of your foot on the inner thigh of your straight leg, with your knee opening out to the side and resting on the ground.

3. Turn your body just a little, so that your heart is facing the foot of your straight leg.

4. Flex the foot of your straight leg.

5. Follow steps 4 to 6 for the straight-leg forward bend pose. (See illustration 13.)

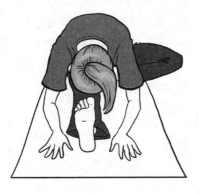

Illustration 13: Head-to-knee pose

Follow-up: Once your child becomes comfortable with these poses, a wonderful way to deepen the energetic experience is to use the breath in coordination with the movement. This significantly increases the calming effect of the movement. Encourage your child to inhale as he gets long, and then exhale when he relaxes down toward the ground. Then once he is in the pose, encourage him to focus on long, slow exhalations (Langhana Breath, in chapter 5, is a great practice to coordinate with this pose).

Challenges: Many children have tightness in their hips and the backs of their legs, and this will often cause them to collapse their torso and round their back as soon as they sit down. For some kids, just sitting up straight is going to be a big challenge! If your child tends to round his back during these poses, try having him bend his knees slightly in the straight-leg variation, and work first on sitting up straight and holding that position for a few breaths. Once that becomes less challenging, you can start working on folding forward. It doesn't matter at all how far you can fold in these poses. It's more important to keep your spine long; the goal is to stretch the back of your body, not to get close to the ground.

Daily Practice: Any of these forward bends are deeply calming, particularly in coordination with the breath. Teach your child that if he is feeling overwhelmed, or notices that he has too much energy for whatever situation he's in, this is a practice he can use to settle his energy.

Strength: Warrior Poses

The warriors are a group of poses that are among the most loved and frequently practiced in adult yoga classes. They all, in slightly different ways, create strength in both the body and the mind. In a graceful metaphor for our own inner strength, these poses rely on flexibility, balance, and patience to build strength, rather than sheer force of body or will.

Warrior 1 Pose

1. Stand in mountain pose (see earlier in this chapter) at the top of your mat. Take a big step back with your left leg.

2. Check out your back foot. It should be completely flat on the ground, with your toes pointing slightly out to the left side.

3. Bend your front knee until it is lined up over your ankle.

4. Face your hips straight ahead.

5. Keeping your legs steady, lift your upper body tall. Now reach your arms straight out in front of your heart. Roll your shoulders back and down.

6. Keeping your arms straight and strong, lift your chest and your arms so that they are pointing toward the ceiling.

7. Look out past your fingertips. Take a few full breaths. (See illustration 14.)

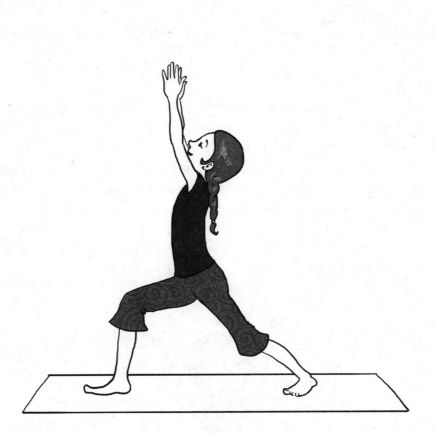

Illustration 14: Warrior 1 pose

8. Relax your arms, step forward into mountain pose, and repeat on the other side.

Warrior 2 Pose

1. Follow steps 1 through 3 for the warrior 1 pose.

2. Instead of turning your hips to face the front, open them up so that your torso is turned to your left side.

3. Open your arms so that your right arm is straight out over your right leg (and parallel to the ground) and your left arm is extended behind you. Your arms should be straight and strong, with your fingertips extended.

4. Gaze out past your front fingertips and take several slow and steady breaths. (See illustration 15.)

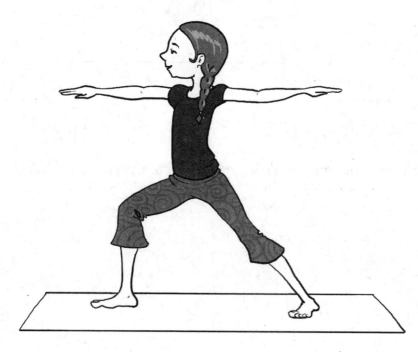

Illustration 15: Warrior 2 pose

5. Relax your arms, step forward into mountain pose, and repeat on the other side.

Warrior 3 Pose

1. Follow steps 1 through 4 for the warrior 1 pose.

2. You are about to come into a balancing variation of warrior, so you will want to find a steady place to fix your gaze first. Look straight ahead of you, and focus on a single thing that isn't moving. It could be a corner of a window, a smudge on the wall, a picture. Anything at all will work.

3. Keep your gaze steady on this spot, and then slowly shift your weight forward, lifting your back leg, tilting your torso forward, and straightening your front leg. Keep the toes of your back leg pointing straight down.

4. There are two different options here for your arms. You can reach them back so that they are parallel to the ground and reaching toward your elevated foot, or you can extend them out past the top of your head (this will be more challenging). Either way, keep your fingers strong and your arms straight. As you come into this pose, try to keep your spine straight and long. Imagine reaching the top of your head forward and the heel of your lifted foot back.

5. If you are feeling very balanced today, you can work on lifting your back leg until it is parallel with the ground (your torso will be parallel to the ground also). This is a challenging pose. Don't worry if you can only lift your leg a little bit while you are learning it! Your body is still getting stronger, and you are still practicing the pose. (See illustration 16.)

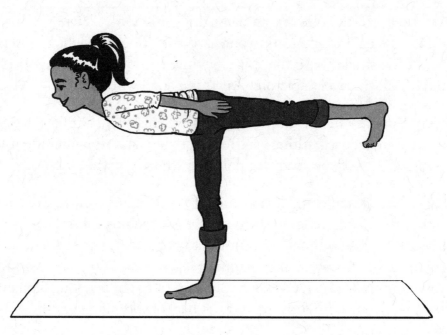

Illustration 16: Warrior 3 pose

6. Breathe slowly in warrior 3, and when you feel like you are ready to move to the other side, slowly bend your front knee and lower your leg back down into warrior 1. Pause for a moment, step forward into mountain pose, and then try the other side.

Follow-up: A favorite activity for many children is to combine the warrior poses with a mantra. A great way to do this is to have a conversation with your child about what a warrior is and the qualities that you need to have in order to be a good warrior. I like to focus the conversation on the ways that you can fight for what is important without hurting anyone else. Choose three qualities that you think are important for a warrior (strength, patience, courage, compassion, etc.). Assign one quality to each warrior pose. Your mantras will be based on these qualities. For example, if you've chosen courage as a quality, you might say, "I have courage" or "I am courageous." Once you've created your three mantras, practice all three warrior poses, moving directly from one to another while saying your mantra for each in a strong voice. If you and your child are practicing these poses together, a wonderful experience for the second side of your poses is to change the beginning of your mantras, so that instead of saying, "I have courage," you would look each other in the eye and say, "You have courage."

Challenges: Many people struggle with the balance of warrior 3. Make sure your child knows that it doesn't matter how high she lifts her back leg, or how long she holds the pose. The important thing is that she practice feeling calm and steady in the pose, and that each time she tries she will get a little stronger and be able to hold her balance a little bit longer.

Daily Practice: While we aren't always in a position to just come into a warrior pose when we need to feel strong, a very good option for times when your child needs a boost is to tell her to visualize herself in her warrior poses, silently repeating her mantra.

Strength: Moving Lunges

Lunges are a simple way to build a lot of strength in the body. In this version we coordinate movement with breathing to deepen the experience and make it more engaging, as well as to increase the strength-building potential.

1. Start in mountain pose (see earlier in this chapter). Lift your right knee up off of the ground and pause for a moment to find your balance.

2. Now take a big step backward and place your right foot on the floor. Your toes should still be pointing straight ahead, with your heel lifted off of the ground.

3. Bend your front knee deeply (make sure not to bend your knee past your ankle).

4. Keeping your legs steady, reach your arms strongly overhead with your fingers extended.

5. Check to see if you are leaning forward a little bit, and if you are, straighten your torso so that it is perpendicular to the ground. Now you are in a lunge. (See illustration 17.)

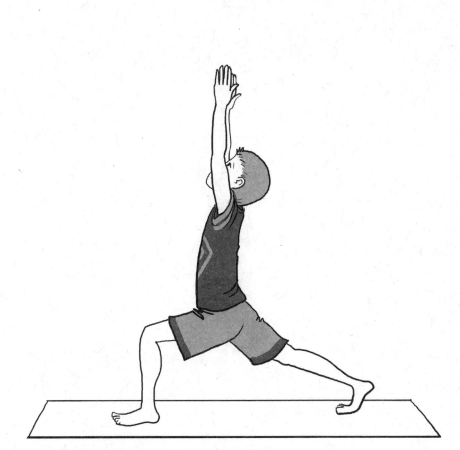

Illustration 17: One posture in the moving lunges series

6. Take a couple of full breaths here in your lunge.

7. The next time you inhale, slowly straighten your front leg while continuing to reach up with your arms. As you straighten your leg, allow your back heel to lift a little higher off of the ground. (See illustration 18.)

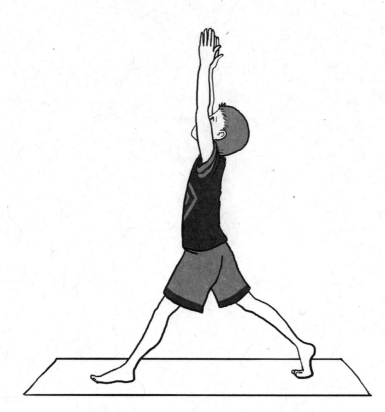

Illustration 18: Another posture in the moving lunges series

8. When it's time to exhale, slowly bend your front knee and press your back heel away from you, lowering your torso straight down.

9. Continue lifting up on your inhale and lowering down on your exhale. Try to keep your upper body moving straight up and down as you bend and straighten your legs, rather than letting it sway forward and backward.

10. Once you get the hang of moving in your lunge, challenge yourself to move up and down for eight full breaths.

11. Step forward and repeat on the other side.

Follow-up: This activity really uses the strength in your legs. After practicing, it will feel great to finish with either bound-ankle pose or head-to-knee pose.

Challenges: Many children and adults find that their balance is tested along with their strength in moving lunges. If your child struggles with his balance during this activity, encourage him to find a focal point to keep his gaze fixed to. It can also be helpful to imagine squeezing your thighs together to activate the small stabilizing muscles in your legs.

Daily Practice: At any time, your child can practice some mindful walking lunges as he moves from place to place. Take a big step forward, and as you breathe out, bend your front knee and lower down into a lunge. Then inhale back up, step your other foot forward, and repeat.

Strength: Boat Pose

Boat pose is a seated posture that uses the entire body. It builds core strength and also necessitates finding a balance between strength and flexibility.

1. Start seated in the middle of your yoga mat. Bend your knees so that your feet are flat on the ground.

2. Sit up very tall and relax your shoulders.

3. Lightly hold on to the backs of your thighs with your hands.

4. Engage your core muscles by pulling your belly button in just a bit, and then lift your feet off of the ground, bringing your shins parallel to the ground.

5. Find your balance and take a few full breaths, using each inhalation to sit up a little bit taller.

6. If this feels good, you may want to try slowly straightening your legs. Once you feel steady, try letting go of your legs and reaching your arms straight out in front of you. (See illustration 19.)

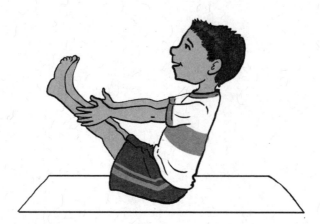

Illustration 19: Boat pose

7. After balancing for a few breaths, or as long as feels good, return to sitting.

Follow-up: Once your child becomes comfortable with boat pose, it can be a lot of fun to play a game called Boat Pose Ball Pass. This game works the core muscles in different ways and also is a great way to practice coordination and cooperation. The basic premise is that a ball is passed from one participant to another with their feet. If you have three or more people to play with, try sitting in a circle and sending the ball around the circle first in one direction, then the other. It's particularly fun to do this to music and challenge yourselves to keep the ball off of the ground for a whole song. If it's just you and your child, you can sit side by side and pass the ball, then turn around and pass it back, so that you are using both sides of your body.

Another great way to make boat pose more interesting is to practice partner boat pose. Sit facing your child, with both of your knees bent and the balls of your feet touching. Reach out and hold hands, then slowly lift your legs up, pressing your feet together. Once both feet are off the ground, take a few breaths together and then slowly lower them down.

Challenges: Some children struggle with the flexibility needed for this pose. If your child is having a hard time, work on lifting her legs to different heights. Encourage her to notice that when her legs are closer to the ground, she has to use more strength, and when they are lifted higher she has to use more flexibility. Try practicing a few seated forward bends right before trying boat pose and see if it feels different.

Daily Practice: While you probably won't practice the full boat pose posture every day, each time you sit down in a chair, try leaning back slightly (without leaning on the back-rest) and lifting your feet just a bit off of the floor. With just this small movement each day, you'll quickly start to develop more core strength.

Balance: Tree Pose

Tree pose is among the most recognizable of yoga poses for a good reason. It is a balancing pose that is both challenging and achievable, and once you've practiced a bit the feeling of steadily grounding down and reaching up at the same time is very satisfying.

1. Begin standing in mountain pose on your yoga mat.

2. Find a place to rest your gaze that is straight out in front of you. Keep staring at that spot throughout the entire practice.

3. Slowly lift your right foot up off of the ground. Bend your knee and turn it out to the side, so that you can place the sole of your right foot on the inside of your left calf.

4. Try to relax the foot of your standing leg. Notice if you are curling up your toes, and if so wiggle them a little to help them relax. Imagine your standing leg growing roots deep into the ground to hold you steady.

5. Press your right foot into your leg, and your leg back into your foot.

6. Bring your hands together in front of your heart. Pause for a moment and then lift them strongly up overhead. You can keep your hands together, or open your arms like branches.

7. As your standing leg grounds down into the earth, imagine your whole body lifting up toward the sky.

8. When you are ready to switch sides, turn your right knee to the front, pause, and then slowly lower it down. Then practice tree pose with your left leg.

Follow-up: Once you have introduced your child to tree pose, and he has had the experience of finding his balance, you can introduce him to a more challenging variation by having him lift his foot higher up onto the inside of his thigh instead of his calf. Make sure to avoid having him place his foot on his knee, which can lead to injury.

Challenges: If this is your child's first experience with a standing balance pose, it might be very frustrating. Some children try to hold their balance by hopping up and down in the pose. Encourage your child to keep staring at his focal point, and if he feels like he is losing his balance, just tell him to place his foot down on the floor, take a full breath in and out, and then pick it back up again.

Daily Practice: One of the great things about tree pose is that it can be practiced anytime you are just standing around. One of my favorite daily rituals is to brush my teeth in tree pose. This is a true challenge, as you are coordinating the balance and focus of tree pose with the movement of your arm and hand. Encourage your child to try brushing on one leg and flossing on the other.

Balance: Side Plank Pose

Side plank is a difficult pose that kids tend to really enjoy. In addition to being a balance, it also builds strength in the arms and the core, and the many variations allow for a progressively more challenging experience.

1. Start on your hands and knees in the center of your mat. Spread your fingers wide and make sure that your whole hand is down on your mat, and that your shoulders are right over your wrists.

2. Now step your feet back so that you are at the top of a push-up position. Press your heels back like you are trying to reach the wall behind you with them. This is called plank pose. Just practicing plank is a great way to build strength through your whole body, but we are going to go a little bit further with the pose.

3. Once you feel steady in plank, shift your weight onto your right hand, and turn your right foot so that the outside edge is on the mat. Very slowly and with careful control, roll your body to the right so that your left leg comes on top of your right leg, and your left arm comes off of the ground. Reach your left arm straight up in the air. This is a basic side plank pose. (See illustration 20.)

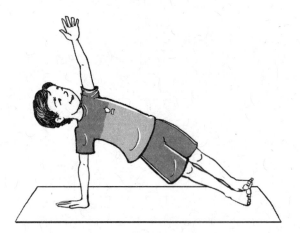

Illustration 20: Side plank pose

4. If you want to give yourself a little extra support, you can use your left leg like a tripod—bend your left knee and place your left foot on the floor in front of your right knee.

5. Try to keep your body in one straight line during this pose. Reach your head in one direction and press your heels in the other. If your hips start to drop, lift them up so that they are in line with the rest of your body. Keep your top arm straight and strong with your fingers extended.

6. When you are ready to switch sides, lower back to plank pose with control, and then either go straight into the other side, or take a rest in child's pose (see illustration 8) between sides.

Follow-up: Side plank is challenging, but if your child loves it and seems ready to go even further, you can try one of the following variations:

- *Lift your top leg straight up off of your bottom leg so your feet are about 2 to 3 feet apart.*

- *Bring your top leg into a tree pose shape (see previous pose), bending at your knee, opening your hip, and placing your foot on either your calf or thigh.*

Challenges: This is a difficult pose that may take some time and practice to feel comfortable. If your child's hips sag or she feels shaky, encourage her to use the tripod-leg variation described above. It's also important to make sure her shoulder is directly over her wrist and that her leg muscles are engaged. The best way to ensure that her legs are engaged is by reminding her to flex her feet.

Daily Practice: This pose is not recommended for daily practice—try it once or twice a week when you have time to focus and work hard.

Balance: Flower Pose

Flower pose is a seated posture that is very accessible. It is both grounding and uplifting, bringing balance to the physical body and to the emotions.

1. Start seated in the middle of your mat.

2. Bring the soles of your feet together and your knees out to the sides. Now separate your feet about ten inches (the outside edges of your feet will stay on the ground).

3. Lean forward just a little, reach your hands in between your knees, and thread your hands and arms under your knees.

4. Turn your palms to face up.

5. Take a full breath in and, as you do, lean back just a little, bringing your feet up off of the ground. Your calves will be resting on your forearms.

6. As you take several breaths here, sit up tall and pull your shoulders back. Spread your fingers wide. You'll know that you have found your balance when the pose feels comfortable and your legs feel light on your arms. (See illustration 21.)

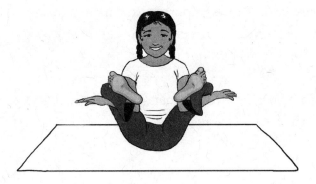

Illustration 21: Flower pose

7. When you are ready to come down, a great way to do it is to unthread your arms, give your knees a squeeze, and slowly lower all the way down onto your back for a rest.

Follow-up: If your child enjoys this pose, and you want to create a longer and more challenging experience, you can try what I call blossoming flower pose. Once you are balanced in flower, unwind your arms (while keeping your legs lifted). Then hold on to the outside edges of your feet and slowly stretch your legs out into a V. Balance there for a few breaths, then bring your legs together into boat pose (see illustration 19).

Challenges: Some children (and adults) tend to let the weight of their legs fall onto their arms during this pose, and it causes them to slouch forward and feel as if they are wrestling their legs into place. It isn't the strength of your arms that lifts your legs in flower pose rather, it is the fact that you shift your weight back and find your balance. Your legs should just lightly rest on your arms. But if your child seems to be slouching, try having him practice boat pose (see illustration 19) directly before flower pose to feel the activation of his core muscles. Then encourage him to try bringing his legs into the shape of flower pose without his arms to get a feel for it before trying again.

Daily Practice: If flower pose feels good to your child, and he has practiced enough to feel steady in it, it can be a great activity to do for a few breaths right before homework or any other activity that requires concentration. The combination of grounding and uplifting feelings is very balancing and contributes to a calm capacity for focus.

Balance: Half Moon Pose

This standing balance is probably the most challenging pose you will practice with your child, and it is also one that children often love. Half moon pose asks you to open yourself up and reach out into the world, and when you find your balance in it, it feels good in the same way that running, jumping, and dancing does. It feels free and light and happy.

1. Begin in warrior 2 pose (see illustration 15).

2. Focus your eyes on a spot on the ground, about six to twelve inches in front of your toes. Slowly reach forward toward that spot, bringing your fingertips down onto the ground and lifting your back leg up off of the ground.

3. Your hand will help you with your balance most if it is placed slightly outside of your foot. A good guide is to have your thumb lined up with, and about six to twelve inches in front of, your pinkie toe. (Your fingers should touch the ground directly below your shoulder.)

4. Now reach your top arm straight up, with your fingers reaching strongly toward the sky.

5. As you find your balance, work on opening up your hips so that they are stacked over each other in a straight line. Flex the foot of your lifted leg.

6. When you feel steady, slowly turn your head to face forward and focus on a spot on the wall right in front of you. If that feels good, try turning to look up past your top hand.

7. When you are ready to finish, bend your front knee and slowly lower yourself back into warrior 2 pose. Step forward with your back leg into mountain pose, then step back with the opposite leg into warrior 2 pose again, and repeat on the other side.

Follow-up: This is not a pose that you will feel great in the first time you try it. It is challenging and may take a lot of practice. Reassure your child that each time she tries, she is getting stronger and improving her balance. She doesn't have to lift her leg very high, or hold the pose very long, in order to be doing a great job.

Challenges: This is a very difficult pose that asks you to use your body in a lot of different ways at once. If your child is having a hard time finding the shape of the pose because of the balancing required, it is a great idea to try practicing it at a wall. Bring the long side of your mat right up against a wall. Stand just a few inches away from the wall and move into warrior 2 pose just like you would in the middle of the room. Follow the same steps as above, but allow your body to lean up against the wall for balance. Once you have a little support, you may find that you can open up into the shape of the pose more freely. Once you've felt that shape in your body with some support, it can be much easier to work toward it on your own, without help from the wall.

Another supportive option is to use a block to help bring the ground closer to your child's bottom hand (see illustration 22). The block (or any other firm object) can be placed at whatever height is most helpful. Start with it higher and, as your child gets more familiar with the pose, lower it for a greater challenge.

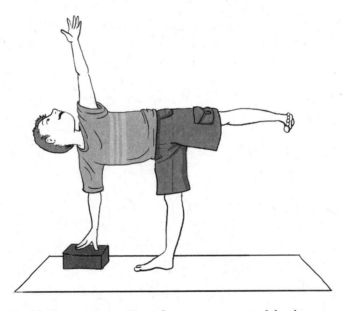

Illustration 22: Half moon pose with a supporting block

Daily Practice: If you have a child that is determined and likes a challenge, working on half moon pose a little bit each day will be very satisfying. It is a pose in which you can really feel your progress if you keep practicing.

Final Relaxation: Savasana

Whether you are practicing just a few poses or a full sequence of all five elements, a wonderful way to end your session is with *savasana*, or "final relaxation." *Savasana* lets the experiences you've had settle into your body and your mind, and provides a transition period that feels nourishing and supportive.

1. Begin seated in the middle of your mat. With your knees bent and your feet on the floor, reach your arms out in between your knees and slowly roll down onto your back.

2. Extend your legs long, and let your feet fall out to the sides.

3. Bring your arms to rest by your sides with your palms facing up.

4. Close your eyes, and let your whole body get heavy and soft.

5. Rest here for as long as you like. You may also want to play some gentle music.

6. When you're ready to get up, do so slowly and gently. Wiggle your fingers and toes, turn your head from side to side, give your knees a hug into your body, and slowly roll onto one side and use your hands to help you come up to sitting.

Follow-up: While it's not always possible to lie down, you can bring the spirit of *savasana* into your body anytime you need a rest. Even if you are seated, try leaning back, closing your eyes, relaxing your muscles, and breathing gently.

Challenges: Some children have a hard time lying flat on their backs. They can feel quite vulnerable and exposed. See chapter 9 for ways to transition into the pose, and also try placing a heavy blanket over your child while in *savasana*.

Daily Practice: *Savasana* is a great follow-up to any yoga pose. Teach it to your child early on in his yoga practice, and encourage him to use it anytime he needs a rest.

Creating a Movement Experience for Your Child

While any of the poses in this chapter can be practiced individually, combining poses into short sequences during your regular practice times will give your child an opportunity to have a more complete energetic experience. When you practice multiple poses at a time, it can be helpful to think about creating a simple energetic bell curve for your child. Start with a calm posture that feels comfortable, then move on to more energizing and challenging poses, and then work your way back to something that feels calming. You can combine any of the poses on your own, but for some suggestions see chapter 9, Putting It All Together.

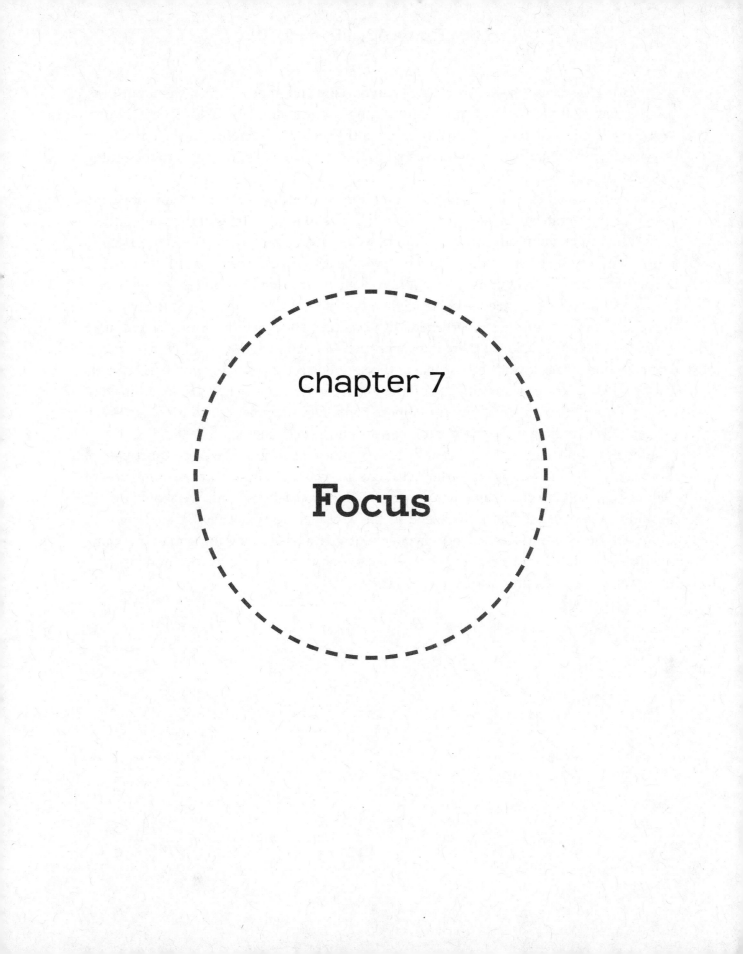

chapter 7

Focus

Learning to focus is a skill that we all can develop and improve throughout our lives, but few of us receive any formal instruction or training in how to do it. For children, improving the ability to focus can make a tremendous difference in their quality of life—everything from their grades in school to their performance in a sport to their interaction with peers is impacted.

As we think about helping our children improve their focus, it's important for us to recognize the significant difference between telling children to focus and teaching them how. When we tell our kids to pay attention, we often assume that what we are asking is reasonable, and that if they don't do what we ask it's because they aren't listening. We think that a lack of attention is a behavior problem, when usually a child is doing the best he can. What kids often need is not discipline but support. As we discussed in chapter 1, the ability to focus can be strengthened with practice, and it will be strengthened more effectively and more rapidly if there is a supportive adult consistently sending the message that the child is safe, loved, and capable of success. The practices of the previous chapters will also help prepare your child to practice focusing. By helping him balance his emotions, reduce stress and anxiety, and feel more confident, the practices all make accessing the thoughtful brain a little easier and focusing a little more manageable.

Children (and many adults) naturally have wandering minds. The constant stream of thoughts, ideas, and feelings that the mind churns out combine with the stimulation of the external world to create an environment in which focusing is hard. We should expect our kids to be distracted, and they need to know that there isn't something wrong with them because focusing is a challenge. Even adults have a hard time tuning in to one thing at a time. The important thing to learn is how to quickly notice when your mind is starting to wander and then to bring it back to the task at hand.

The Practices

The activities in this chapter offer a variety of options for giving your child something concrete to practice focusing on. The goal of each activity is for her to notice when her mind is wandering and then bring it back to the object of focus, strengthening her capacity to regain her focus in daily life.

When you start exploring these activities with your child, start with short increments of time (often even one to two minutes is a good start), and increase the time slowly, letting your child know that the time increase might be challenging. Practicing in a calm, quiet space with minimal outside distractions will help while your child is first learning these activities. As her capacity for focus increases, practicing in a space where life is happening around her will be a challenge that helps your child begin to use the tools she is learning in a real-world context.

Most meditation practices are traditionally done in a seated position. Sitting has some advantages. You can be relaxed while sitting, but you're unlikely to fall asleep, which is a real possibility if you choose to do these activities lying down. It you are practicing Focus activities as part of a longer yoga session, the best option is usually to have your child sit upright on her yoga mat. If sitting in a cross-legged position is uncomfortable or distracting for your child, it's no problem to use a chair.

Exploring Your Drishti

"*Drishti*" is a Sanskrit word that means "focal point." During yoga practice, finding and maintaining a *drishti* is an important part of learning steadiness during balancing poses, and practicing finding your *drishti* during movement is a great preparation for the seated meditation activities that we will practice next. In this activity, we're going to use tree pose to practice maintaining an external *drishti*.

1. Review tree pose in chapter 6. You are going to practice tree pose several times, changing your *drishti* each time while noticing how it affects the pose.

2. In the first version of tree pose, give yourself a very clear, specific place to keep your eyes focused. You can try placing an object like a small stone out on the ground in front of you, or you can put a sticker on the wall opposite your mat. Focus on your object even before you lift your foot off of the ground. Notice how your body feels with this fixed *drishti*, and also notice what happens if your eyes wander off of your *drishti* for a moment. If this happens, just see what it feels like, and then bring your eyes back to your *drishti*. Don't switch legs yet.

3. In the second version of tree pose that you are going to explore, try standing in front of a window and gazing outside, balancing on the same leg as in step 2. Allow your eyes to take in the whole scene in front of you, and notice how your body feels.

4. Next, try the most challenging version of all. Practice tree pose with your eyes closed! If you feel very wobbly, just put your foot down and pick it back up again. Notice what it feels like in your body and how it affects your balance when your eyes are closed.

5. After you have tried each version of tree pose, practice on the other side. When you balance on the opposite leg, first try with your eyes closed, then looking out a window, and finally with a fixed *drishti*.

Follow-up: Talk with your child about his experience in each of the variations. Next time you practice tree pose, remind him about his *drishti*. In tree pose, when your mind starts to wander, your eyes usually do as well, and losing your balance is your body's reminder to stay focused.

Challenges: Balancing poses are hard, even when you are focused on a *drishti*. Sometimes when your child feels that he is losing his balance, he might begin to hop up and down to maintain it. Encourage him instead to just put his foot down, take a breath, refocus, and start again.

Daily Practice: There are many situations in daily life when you need to find your balance, particularly if you are very active. Encourage your child to begin noticing all of the times that he would benefit from better balance—such as before a soccer game or gymnastics practice, when carrying something heavy or awkward, or even while waiting in line or sitting still for extended periods. Then ask him to experiment with finding a steady *drishti* during those moments. It's likely that with practice he will discover the grounding benefits of a *drishti* and incorporate it into his routines.

Expanding-Energy Meditation

This meditation is a favorite for many children. When you are really focusing in on the practice, it is an exciting way to feel the energy that makes up the entire natural world (including us) right in your hands. This activity offers such a concrete way to know if your mind is wandering. As soon as you take your mind off of the meditation, you won't be able to feel the energy in your hands!

1. Sit on your mat, with your body tall and relaxed. Take a few full breaths to settle your body and your mind, and then close your eyes.

2. Bring your hands together and begin to rub your palms vigorously. Continue to rub faster and faster until your hands feel warm, then slowly stop rubbing and keep your palms together.

3. Imagine that between your hands is a very tiny but very bright and strong ball of light and energy. As you take a full breath in, very, very slowly separate your hands and imagine that ball of light growing and expanding, filling your hands with energy. (If you are modeling this for your child, let your hands come to about the width of your body.) (See illustration 23.)

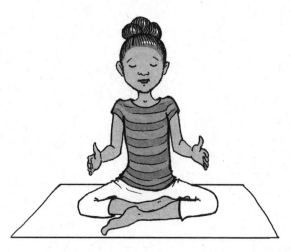

Illustration 23: Expanding-energy meditation

4. When you are ready to breathe out, gently and slowly push your hands back together, squeezing that ball of light until it gets very small.

5. Continue expanding your energy ball as you breathe in and squeezing it together as you breathe out, keeping the rest of your body as still as you can.

6. Try practicing Expanding-Energy Meditation for about two minutes the first time you try it, and then a little bit longer each time after that.

Follow-up: When you finish this meditation, ask your child what she felt. Often she will be completely shocked at how strongly she could feel the energy in her hands. Common responses are that her hands felt warm, that it felt like there were magnets pulling them together, that they felt tingly, and that the ball got heavier and heavier.

Challenges: If your child (or you) is having trouble feeling the energy in her hands, don't worry! When we aren't used to feeling something it can take a little bit of time to find it. Every once in a while children say that they couldn't feel anything during this practice; this is a typical response when they moved their hands too quickly or separated them too far during the exercise. It should take the entire length of your inhalation to bring your hands apart, and they should end up about body width. It should also take the entire length of your exhalation to push them back together. Some children need to practice for a little bit longer to start feeling the energy, so if your child agrees, try again for three or four minutes and see how it goes. Make sure that you aren't pressuring your child to feel something that she doesn't feel. Try to avoid making suggestions about what she might be feeling, or she may start to feel like she is doing something wrong.

Daily Practice: While Expanding-Energy Meditation will usually be practiced during a yoga session, if your child seems to connect with this practice you might suggest that she try it anytime she feels disconnected from the world around her.

Single-Pointed Focus

A very simple but effective type of meditation is the practice of fixing your gaze on one steady object for a set period of time. You may have heard of an adult practice of fixing one's gaze on a candle flame. With children we get more creative to find safer variations of the practice.

1. Choose something to be the object of your gaze. This is an important choice. A candle flame works so well for an adult practice because it is at once constant and ever changing. A candle flame has a small amount of movement that keeps drawing you in, but it doesn't change so much that it inspires thoughts or ideas. Try to choose something with similar qualities for your practice with your child: a sand timer, a jar filled with water and glitter that you can shake, a battery-operated flickering candle (try putting it inside a brown paper bag), or something out in nature such as a stream, clouds changing shape, or leaves moving in the wind. Involving your child in this choice will make the entire practice more interesting to him.

2. Sit down on your yoga mat with your chosen object in front of you. If you are outside using an object in nature for this practice, make sure you have something clean and comfortable to sit on. Sit up tall and take a few full breaths to prepare.

3. Set a timer for two minutes (this is a good amount of time to start with, but you can try more or less depending on your child's prior capacity and experience).

4. Fix your gaze on the object you've chosen, and let it fill up your mind.

5. Now, here is the most important part of this practice: When your mind wanders away from your object, try to notice right away, and then bring it back. The exercise of noticing your mind wandering, and practicing bringing it back, is the true purpose of this activity. Keep practicing until your timer goes off.

6. When the timer goes off, close your eyes and try to keep the object you have been gazing at fixed in your mind. Take a few full breaths, and when you are ready open your eyes.

Follow-up: Talk with your child about his experience practicing Single-Pointed Focus. Allow him time to share whether he was able to notice his mind wandering, and even what his mind wandered to. Practicing this alongside your child, and sharing some thoughts about your own wandering mind, is a helpful part of the experience. As your child gets more comfortable with this practice, extend the amount of time on the timer.

Challenges: Some children feel frustrated when they notice their mind wandering. They think that the point of the practice is to stay connected to their object for the whole time they are practicing, and that if their mind wanders they are doing something wrong. Make sure your child knows that everyone's mind wanders. It is the job of his mind to make thoughts, and that is a good thing! Remind him that this activity is about noticing when his mind wanders, and that every time he notices his mind wandering he is doing the activity perfectly.

Daily Practice: Learning to notice when your mind wanders, and bring it back to the activity you want to be focusing on, is a vital life skill. Your child can remind himself of this practice anytime he has something important to do. Encourage him to take a few full breaths before starting, and remind him that it is totally natural for his mind to wander. Whether he is trying to focus on homework, a test, learning a song on the piano, or listening to a friend talk, his mind will still keep making thoughts. The important thing is that he can recognize when his mind is wandering, and bring it back.

Thought River Meditation

This seated meditation practice begins to introduce your child (in a more concrete way) to the idea of nonjudgmental awareness of her thoughts and ideas.

1. Start by having a brief discussion with your child. Ask her if she ever has lots of thoughts and ideas floating around in her head. Ask her if she ever gets stuck paying attention to one of those thoughts when she doesn't want to (you can use the example of a song being stuck in your head). Now introduce the idea that our minds are like thought machines. It's the job of your mind to make thoughts all the time, but we get to decide if we are going to listen to them, and we get to decide if we are going to believe them. Now is a good time to introduce the idea that you don't have to believe everything that you think! Let her know that even though the mind makes thoughts all the time, we get to choose whether we want to spend time thinking about those thoughts. It's important that your child understands that there is nothing wrong with her for having lots of thoughts—it actually means her mind is working perfectly. In this discussion, introduce the idea of imagining a river of thoughts flowing by us. Our minds are constantly making new thoughts and dropping them into this river. We see the thoughts float by, and when we notice them we have a choice. We can either pick them up and explore them (think about them!), or we can just notice them and then let them go floating by.

2. Tell your child that, for a few minutes, you are going to practice letting your thoughts drift by on that river. Answer any questions that she has before you begin. Make sure you let your child know that having lots of thoughts isn't bad—it just means that she has a strong mind and it's working hard.

3. Find a comfortable position to sit in. When our bodies are uncomfortable, we get distracted from our thoughts.

4. Close your eyes and picture a river flowing right past you. As thoughts begin to pop into your head, imagine placing those thoughts gently on the river to float downstream.

5. After a few minutes, ring a singing bowl to signal to your child that she should open her eyes.

6. Take some time to talk with your child about her experience.

Follow-up: A wonderful follow-up to this practice is to do an art project, during which you take some time to draw your river of thoughts. Try practicing this alongside your child, and see if drawing together inspires some conversation (but don't worry if it doesn't—just sharing the experience is worthwhile).

Challenges: The first few times you practice this activity, you might find that you are thinking about thinking. Thoughts such as "What am I thinking about now?" or "I don't think I'm thinking anything" are common and can go into the river just like every other thought. Children often ask if a feeling or sensation is a thought. If you feel something (like an itch), that's a sensation, but as soon as your mind says to itself "Oh, that itches," then you're having a thought! Try to practice long enough to let that initial mental chatter about the activity itself fall away. Your child may say that she didn't have any thoughts, or that she couldn't put them in the river. It's worth continuing to practice this activity even if those things come up. It may take several sessions of talking about these ideas in order for your child to start feeling that she is actually having the experience.

Daily Practice: Thought River Meditation can be practiced anytime you are feeling overwhelmed or are having a hard time focusing. Let your child know that she can close her eyes for a moment or two, let her thoughts float down the river, and give herself a rest from her mental chatter.

Focusing in Daily Life

As your child learns that bringing his mind back to the task at hand is a skill, he will find lots of opportunities to practice it in daily life. Just like the mind wants to wander during Focus activities, the mind wants to wander during homework, test taking, instrument practice, and even during conversations with you! Remember that the wandering mind is natural, and rather than becoming angry or frustrated, just remind your child that he is perfectly capable of noticing his wandering mind, taking a full breath, and bringing his attention back to the task at hand.

If your child is having a particularly challenging day, or will be called upon to exert a large amount of focus in an upcoming activity, it can be useful to give him a little bit of time for a mind-wander break. This is just a defined stretch of time during which he is free to daydream and let his mind go anywhere it wants. I recommend setting a timer for mind-wander breaks. In order to truly give your mind a wander break, you will want to avoid conversation and outside stimulation such as music or television.

When you are interacting with your child, notice if your own mind starts to wander at any point. Kids have an almost uncanny ability to sense when our attention is diverted or fragmented. If your mind wanders when you are talking with your child, and you think he has noticed, let him know that you realized your mind was wandering, caught it, brought it back, and that he now has your full attention.

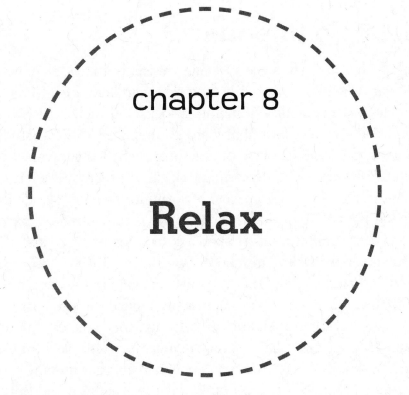

chapter 8

Relax

In order for any person, a child or an adult, to be the best version of him- or herself, he or she must get enough sleep. Think about yourself on a day when you are exhausted. Are you as nice to other people? As capable of making good decisions? Able to maintain your focus and get things done efficiently? Because their brains are still developing, children who are exhausted suffer even more than we do, yet the majority of kids in the United States aren't getting enough sleep.

In this final step of our yoga and mindfulness practice, we will learn activities that help children rest and restore, reduce insomnia, and help with the transition to sleep.

Why Is Rest So Important?

Sleep among children has been the subject of many research studies, all of which conclude the same thing—that even a small amount of lost sleep can dramatically impact children's school success, including their ability to maintain focus and their ability to store memories. Impulse control and emotional stability are also reduced. A 2003 study found that one hour of lost sleep (during the course of just three nights) is equivalent to the loss of two years of cognitive development—meaning that the sixth-grade students in the study who were getting just a little bit less sleep were performing at a fourth-grade level in school (Sadeh, Gruber, and Raviv 2003)! Another fascinating study of more than seven thousand high school students in Minnesota showed a correlation between just fifteen minutes less sleep and a full grade point drop in school (Wahlstrom 2010).

These types of findings are replicated over and over again in the academic research on sleep among children and teens. Sleep loss appears to reduce the strength of our prefrontal cortex (the Thoughtful Brain). Among other things, this reduces children's ability to focus well, particularly on things that are challenging. Sleep also plays an important role in storing memories—when children don't get enough sleep, they literally can't remember what they are learning (Aton, Seibt, and Frank 2009; Diekelmann and Born 2010).

There are also emotional consequences to reduced sleep among children. Being tired, for both kids and adults, often leads to irritability, anger, a shortened temper, and reduced compassion for others. Stressful things feel more stressful, and it gets harder to see the bright side of life. Judgment is impaired, impulse control is reduced, and behavior gets worse. Many tired children show an increase in hyperactive behavior and are quick to become overstimulated. Lack of sleep is correlated with an increase in ADHD symptoms and, in some cases, can even lead to behavior that gets misdiagnosed as ADHD.

What Can We Do to Help?

The National Sleep Foundation recommends that children between five and twelve years old get ten to twelve hours of sleep each night. Most children get far less, even though most parents think their kids are getting enough sleep. The reasons why children have trouble falling asleep and staying asleep are many: stress and anxiety, overscheduling, early school start times, too much homework, noise and lights from urban environments or loud households, and many more. While some factors affecting your child's sleep quantity and quality can be addressed directly (earlier bedtime, black-out shades), and some can't be helped at all (school start time), reducing your child's stress level will help improve her quality of sleep, and teaching her relaxing activities that she can use to quiet her mind and transition to sleep will help her actually fall asleep when she goes to bed.

The Practices

The activities in this chapter are based on restorative yoga practices that provide profound relaxation for both the body and the mind. In restorative yoga, the idea is to set your body up in a particular pose where it is well supported, and then completely relax, allowing gravity to do all of the work. These poses are held for an extended length of time based what feels good. When you practice these poses with your child, try to create a space that feels nurturing, safe, and calm. Dim light and gentle music can be very supportive. For many children, using a blanket over the whole body during restorative poses is deeply soothing and creates an increased feeling of safety. If your child responds better to one of these activities in particular, it's a good idea to keep using it. Don't worry about varying the activities, particularly if your child is practicing before bedtime. Practicing the same Relax activity each day will only deepen its impact as the body learns to settle down more quickly.

Legs Up the Wall Pose

This restorative yoga pose is a favorite of both children and adults. It is simple to do but has a powerfully relaxing effect on both the body and the mind.

1. Set up your yoga mat so that the short end is against a wall (one that is free of hanging photos or other obstructions).

2. The easiest way to get into this pose is to come into child's pose (see illustration 8) just off to one side of your yoga mat, with your feet and hips very close to the wall and the top of your head facing the center of the room. Then slowly roll over onto your back, extending your legs up the wall as you go.

3. Once there you may need to scoot yourself in so that your legs are flush to the wall. If the backs of your legs are especially tight, then move a bit away from the wall until your legs feel comfortable.

4. You can rest here with your arms by your sides, palms face up (see illustration 24), or bring one hand to your heart and one to your belly. This is an excellent place to practice Heart and Belly Breath (see chapter 5).

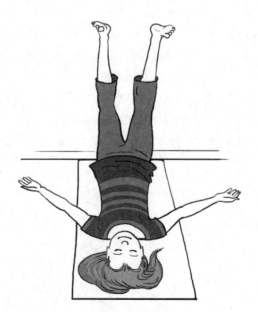

Illustration 24: Legs up the wall pose

5. Rest in this pose for at least three minutes, although you can stay here for as long as ten or fifteen minutes if you feel comfortable.

6. If you have one available, try using an eye pillow during this pose.

7. When you are ready to come out of the pose, pull your knees into your chest and roll to one side. Then use your hands to come back up to sitting.

Follow-up: A wonderful addition to this pose for your child is a gentle neck, forehead, or hand massage from you! Use some yummy-smelling lotion, and sit behind your child's head. Slide your hands under the back of her neck, and slowly and gently slide one hand and then the other from the base of her neck to the back of her head. Get a rhythm going and alternate hands for a few moments. Then gently place her head on the ground and, using your thumbs, massage her forehead using long strokes from the bridge of her nose to her temples, and follow that same pattern up along her forehead. Then move quietly and slowly to each of her hands and gently massage them. When you are finished with her hands, position yourself behind her head again and rest your hands on her shoulders for a moment to let her know that you are done.

Challenges: Some people have trouble feeling relaxed in this pose, because tightness in the back of their legs makes it hard to rest at the 90-degree angle that the body needs to be in here. If that is the case for your child, make practicing seated forward bends a priority (see chapter 6). Sometimes the legs up the wall pose feels a little awkward, and you might find your legs sliding to one side or into a V shape. If that happens, try changing your position just a little bit—you may need to be a little closer or a little farther away from the wall.

Daily Practice: This is a wonderful pose to practice right before bed (if your bed is against a wall, you can even practice in bed!), especially if you have any trouble falling asleep.

Supported Reclined Bound-Ankle Pose

Reclined bound-ankle pose is a tremendously powerful restorative posture, especially when supported with blankets or bolsters. It provides a deep experience of relaxation and also very gently opens your hips and your upper chest, making breathing a little easier and movement more fluid. This pose is like hitting a reset button for a tired and stiff body.

1. Prepare some props that will help you get most comfortable in this pose. You will want to use two firm blankets or two blocks for under your knees, another blanket or bolster for under your back, an eye mask if you have one, and another blanket to lay over your whole body. If you are using bolsters, place them next to your mat. If you are using blankets, roll one blanket into a short, thick roll, at least eight inches in diameter and about as long as your own back. Fold the other two blankets into squares or rectangles about six inches high (these are approximate measurements—just give this all a try and you'll soon figure out what works best for you). Open up your last blanket completely.

2. Set all of your props next to your yoga mat. Sit with the bottoms of your feet together and your knees open, as in bound-ankle pose (see illustration 12).

3. Put either the bolsters or the folded blankets under your knees so that they are supported.

4. Now bring another bolster or the rolled-up blanket behind you. One short end of the bolster or blanket should be right up against your hips. Slowly lower your body down so that you are lying on top of the blanket or bolster (it should be long enough to support your head; if not, use another blanket or a firm pillow). (See illustration 25.)

5. Pull your last blanket up over your body to keep you warm. If you have an eye mask, lay it over your eyes.

6. Open your arms out to your sides, with your palms facing up (underneath the blanket).

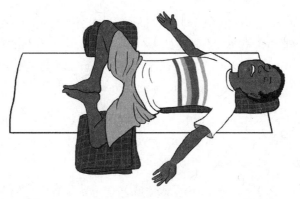

Illustration 25: Supported reclined bound-ankle pose

7. Rest here for as long as you want. The more time you spend here, the more rejuvenated you'll feel when you are finished.

Follow-up: Once this pose becomes comfortable and familiar, a wonderful way to deepen the experience is to practice a Connect, Breathe, or Focus activity while you are resting. Good ones to try are Heart and Belly Breath, Langhana Breath, Layers of Sound, or Thought River Meditation.

Challenges: For most people, this is a very comfortable pose, but for some children tightness in the hips might make holding the pose for an extended period more challenging. If that is the case for your child, try using a bigger bolster or thicker blanket to better support his knees. It doesn't matter how widely they are opened. If, after a minute or two, he is still uncomfortable, encourage him to slowly bring his knees together and extend his legs straight, allowing them to fall open to the sides like in *savasana* (see chapter 6). Finish out the experience in this modified version of the pose.

Daily Practice: Like the pose legs up the wall, this pose is a fantastic tool for children who have a hard time falling asleep at night, and it can also be practiced right in bed. If your child is practicing on a soft mattress, or if you think he might fall asleep in this position, then omit the blanket or bolster behind his back.

Guided Visualization

A guided visualization is an imaginary exploration that you lead your child through. Creating a guided visualization is an exercise in creativity, but it is simple once you get started. Getting comfortable creating visualizations for your child will provide you with a limitless world of options for helping her to relax.

1. Have your child relax in *savasana* (see chapter 6) or sit in a comfortable position. Darkening the room, using an eye mask if you have it, and covering up with a blanket will all deepen the experience of relaxation.

2. Choose a location for your imaginary experience. The most soothing visualizations are usually ones that explore the natural world. Good choices include the beach, the forest, a lake, an open field of flowers, a hillside while it's snowing, or any other location with the potential for a rich sensory experience.

3. Once you've chosen a location for your visualization, you will want to talk your child through an exploration of that locale. For example, you might begin a visualization of a walk through the woods by saying, "Step into the forest, and notice what the leaves underfoot sound like. Take a few more steps, and then reach your hand out to feel the bark of a tree nearby. Does it feel smooth or scratchy or rough? Notice the color of the bark. Take a deep breath in and notice what the forest smells like. . . ."

Some things to keep in mind:

- You are setting the scene for your child, but you want her to have her own experience, so avoid using language that describes her experience with adjectives (for example, avoid saying "notice the wonderful smell of the forest" or "feel the soothing cool breeze on your face"). The smell of the forest might not be so wonderful in your child's mind, and that is absolutely fine. The idea is to open the senses and just experience something new through the mind. When you add qualifying words you create the potential for your child to feel like she is somehow doing this wrong if what she feels isn't the same as what you say.

- Use a quiet voice, but don't fall into the trap of becoming monotonous. Your voice should sound normal, and fluctuations in pacing, pitch, and volume are perfectly fine. Just avoid making your voice substantially louder at any point or you might startle your child.

- Use guiding questions to encourage a full sensory experience, and keep your child engaged. Things like, "Stick out your tongue and catch a snowflake. What does it taste like?" or "Look out at the water. What colors do you see reflected in it?" Make sure when you ask questions, you pause for a few moments before moving on.

4. Pay attention to your child to figure out how long your guided visualizations should be. When you first start, a little bit of fidgeting is normal. You want to keep going long enough to get those first wiggles behind you, but then once she has been calm for a little while, if you start to see her getting fidgety again, it's time to start wrapping up.

5. When you are ready to finish up your visualization, a great way to end is by guiding your child into *savasana* wherever she is in her imagination. Talk her into lying down in the grass or on a warm rock. Then play some soothing music for a few minutes and let her decide when to get up.

Follow-up: Many children love to follow up a guided visualization with an art activity during which they can draw their experience. Others enjoy leading their parents through a visualization of their own creation.

Challenges: There are two potential challenges for your child during a guided visualization. The first is that she falls asleep. This is common in children who are exhausted or aren't sleeping well at night. If your child is falling asleep within the few minutes of this practice, then it's likely that she needs the sleep more than she needs the visualization, and my recommendation is to let her nap. The other challenge is the potential for your child's mind to wander, or for her to become bored. If your child has a wandering mind, keep the actual visualization short, and allow for restful mind-wander time at the end of the practice (see Focus in Daily Life in chapter 7). Follow-up activities like drawing, or even just talking about the experience, will likely keep her more tuned in next time.

Daily Practice: Visualizations are like organized daydreams, and many children find that they quickly learn to create them for themselves. If your child enjoys creating her own guided visualizations, allow her time during the day to take a break. Let her know that any time she needs a mental vacation, she can put a timer on for a few minutes and lead herself on an imaginary adventure.

Tense and Let Go: Yoga Nidra

"Yoga *nidra*" means "yoga sleep," and this is a relaxation practice that is thought to be a state between sleeping and wakefulness, where the practitioner is at complete rest yet still consciously aware. In an adult practice, awareness is brought slowly through each part of the body, relaxing first the physical body, then the mind and the emotions. In this child-appropriate version we are going to use a more direct experience of the body to help make the practice more accessible and engaging.

1. Begin reclined in *savasana* (see chapter 6) on your mat. You can use an eye pillow and a blanket over your body, if they will help you get more comfortable.

2. Spend a few moments here just paying attention to your breath and getting settled.

3. Now you are going to bring your attention to each part of your body, starting with your toes and moving all the way up to your head. As you think about each part of your body, you will tense the muscles in that body part, and then let them relax, until you have invited your whole body to relax.

4. First think about your toes. Scrunch them up as tight as you can, hold them there for a second or two, and then let them rest. Now tense up both of your feet, and when you let them relax, imagine that they are very, very heavy.

5. Now tighten the muscles in your calves and around your knees. Try counting to five before letting them relax.

6. Next squeeze all of the muscles in your legs. You might find yourself squeezing so hard that your legs lift off of the ground a tiny bit. After a few seconds, let all of the muscles in your legs relax, and feel your legs settle comfortably into the ground.

7. Now pull your belly button in for a few seconds, and then let your belly get very soft. Relax your back into the floor.

8. Scrunch your shoulders up to your ears, then after a few seconds relax them down.

9. Make your hands into very tight fists, and squeeze all of the muscles in your arms. Just like your legs, you may find that your arms come off of the ground a little, and that is great. Now relax your arms and your hands, letting them rest by your sides with your palms facing up.

10. Close your eyes very tightly, scrunch up your nose, and squeeze your lips together. Hold your face in this tensed position for a few seconds, and then let your whole face relax. Take a big breath in and, when you exhale, let out a deep sigh through your mouth.

11. Now take a minute to pay attention to your whole body. If you notice any part that still feels uncomfortable or isn't very relaxed, go ahead and tense it up, then let go, until you've relaxed each part of you.

12. Once your body is relaxed, rest in *savasana* for as long as you'd like.

Follow-up: The Tense and Let Go relaxation is a very straightforward activity that has the potential to create a powerful sense of ease and release for your child. Once your child is comfortable with this physical practice, you may want to consider adding a component that asks him if he is having any feelings or thoughts that are keeping him from relaxing. If so, you can practice Thought River Meditation (see chapter 7) as a second part of this activity. Guide your child through a practice of picking his uncomfortable thought up out of the river, holding it tightly for a few seconds, and then putting it back in the river to float away.

Challenges: If your child is struggling with this activity, it is possible that it is just too long for him right now. Feel free to change the language of this practice so that it moves more quickly (for example tensing entire areas of the body at once) or more slowly (as slowly as tensing one toe at a time for some kids) based on the needs of your child.

Daily Practice: Like the other Relax activities, Tense and Let Go is a perfect transition to bedtime for many children. If your child enjoys this practice, encourage him to make it part of his bedtime routine.

Relaxation for Parents

It's entirely likely that you have been sleep deprived from the day your child was born. Making time for your own self-care is crucial to your own capacity for emotional balance, good decision making, and the ability to focus on your child's needs. As you share these Relax activities with your child, go ahead and try them yourself. Set up a short bedtime ritual that helps ease you into sleep. When you feel like you need a nap in the middle of the day but just don't have time for one, try a restorative pose or a short Tense and Let Go practice instead of another cup of coffee.

If you are lucky enough to have a yoga studio nearby that offers restorative yoga classes, sign up immediately. If you can't find a class, I highly recommend *Relax and Renew: Restful Yoga for Stressful Times*, by Judith Lasater.

chapter 9

Putting It All Together

As you begin sharing yoga and mindfulness with your child, remember what we discussed in chapter 3. Start slow, introducing activities with plenty of time for exploration and conversation. Don't pressure yourself or your child to move through activities quickly. There is no checklist and no time frame for your practice.

As you schedule time to work with your child, remember that a combination approach—whereby you have one or two longer sessions per week, combined with reminders to integrate the tools into daily life—is recommended. In your longer sessions, try to incorporate activities from different elements of the practice, even if your child has a strong preference for one or two elements (for example, some kids are happy to practice Move activities and leave out everything else; others would love to do Relax activities for the whole session). Yoga is most powerful as a holistic practice.

Although you should feel free to combine activities in ways that appeal to you and to your child, what follows are some suggestions for sequences based on approximately twenty-, forty-, and sixty-minute practices. When your child is first learning the practices, these sequences will take longer than they might later on, when the activities are more familiar. If you choose to create your own sequences, keep in mind that a useful way to think about a practice session is as a gentle bell curve, whereby you are starting off in a calm place, then working up toward things that are more energetic and challenging, and then ending with something relaxing. Don't worry if you get started on a sequence, decide to dedicate more time than you had planned to a particular activity, and don't get a chance to finish the sequence. If your child is engaged, it's always worth it to spend the time on what he is interested in. Just try to finish up with a relaxing activity and/or a short *savasana*.

This is a good time to review the guidelines in chapter 3, and to choose an opening and closing ritual for your practice sessions.

Recommended Sequences
(All time frames are approximate—don't rush!)

20 minutes	Layers of Sound; Cat, Cow, and Twist Poses; Bound-Ankle Pose; Moving Lunges; Heart and Belly Breath; Tense and Let Go; Savasana
20 minutes	Heart and Belly Breath; Walking Meditation; Mountain Pose; Warrior 1 Pose; Flower Pose; Thought River Meditation; Savasana
20 minutes	Balloon Breath; Tree Pose; Exploring Your Drishti; Straight-Leg Forward Bend; Legs Up the Wall Pose
40 minutes	Heart and Belly Breath; I Am In Charge Mantra; Mountain Pose; Warrior 1 Pose (on one side, with the left leg back); Warrior 3 Pose (on the same side, with the left leg back); Warrior 1 Pose (on the other side, with the right leg back); Warrior 3 pose (on the same side, with the right leg back); Malasana; Bound-Ankle Pose; Expanding-Energy Meditation; Savasana
40 minutes	Layers of Sound; Cat, Cow, and Twist Poses; Head-to-Knee Pose; Warrior 2 Pose (on one side, with the left leg back); Half Moon Pose (on the same side, with the left leg in the air); Mountain Pose; Warrior 2 Pose (on the other side, with the right leg back); Half Moon Pose (on the same side, with the right leg in the air); Walking Meditation; Langhana Breath; Guided Visualization; Savasana
40 minutes	Emotion Jar; Alternate-Nostril Breathing; Cat, Cow, and Twist Poses; Moving Lunges; Boat Pose; Straight-Leg Forward Bend; Caring Feelings; Supported Reclined Bound-Ankle Pose
60 minutes	Checking-In Worksheet; Alternate-Nostril Breathing; Cat, Cow, and Twist Poses; Child's Pose; Mountain Pose; Warrior 1 (on one side, left leg back, with mantra); Warrior 2 (on the same side, left leg back, with mantra); Warrior 3 (on the same side, left leg in the air, with mantra); Warrior 1 (on the other side, right leg back, with mantra); Warrior 2 (on the same side, right leg back, with mantra); Warrior 3 (on the same side, right leg in the air, with mantra); Tree Pose; Malasana; Seated Forward Bend (your choice); Single-Pointed Focus; Supported Reclined Bound-Ankle Pose

60 minutes	Balloon Breath; Cat, Cow, and Twist Poses; Head-to-Knee Forward Bend; Exploring Your Drishti; Warrior 2 (on one side, with the left leg back); Half Moon Pose (on the same side, with left leg back); Warrior 2 (on the other side, with right leg back); Half Moon Pose (on the same side, with right leg in the air); Mountain Pose; Child's Pose; Side Plank Pose; I Am In Charge Mantra; Tense and Let Go; Savasana
60 minutes	Layers of Sound; Back-to-Back Breathing; Straight-Leg Forward Bend; Flower Pose; Boat Pose; Partner Boat Pose; Head-to-Knee Forward Bend; Flower Pose; Straight-Leg Forward Bend; Expanding-Energy Meditation; Legs Up the Wall Pose

Transitions

When you are practicing several activities in one session, an important part of the experience that often gets neglected is the transitions. Sometimes, when you move from one activity to another, you can lose your child's attention as you transition, particularly when moving from sitting to standing or vice versa, or from sitting to reclining. You say "stand up" and your child takes it as an invitation to jump, run in circles, go get a snack, and so on. My recommendation is that you make the transitions part of the experience as much as possible, guiding your child with specific instructions for standing and sitting. The transitions that follow include some possible ways to do this, but you are welcome to get creative and come up with other ways to transition that are enjoyable but specific.

Another instance in which you will want to make deliberate use of transitions is when you feel you need to bring your child's energy level up or down in preparation for what is coming next. Sometimes it's helpful to insert small amounts of stimulating or relaxing movement in between activities so that your child is better prepared.

From Sitting to Standing: No-Hands Stand

This is a fun but challenging way to transition to standing, and while both you and your child may struggle with it at first, keep trying and it will get much easier quickly.

1. From a sitting position, bend your knees and plant your feet on the floor (close to your hips).

2. Reach your arms straight out in front of you between your knees.

3. Use your core strength to shift your weight forward onto your feet and slowly lift up to standing, without putting your hands on the ground.

4. Feel free to rock back and forth to get some momentum going to help lift you up. Try just a little weight shift, or even a full roll onto your back.

From Standing to Sitting: Tiptoe Pose to Squatting

This is another transition that will build core strength while keeping your child engaged and focused.

1. Begin in mountain pose (see chapter 6) with your gaze steady and focused.

2. Stretch your arms out in front of you.

3. Slowly lift up onto the balls of your feet and pause for a moment.

4. On a long, slow exhale, begin to bend your knees (see illustration 26) and come all the way down into a squat. Then, lower to sitting.

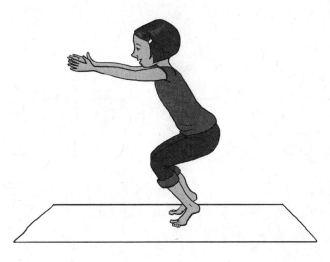

Illustration 26: Going from standing to sitting, or tiptoe pose to squatting

From Sitting to Reclining: Smallest You to Biggest You

Sometimes it's hard to get your child reclined on her back for Relax activities or *savasana*. She may want to curl up on her side, or roll onto her belly, but this transition can help.

1. Sit in the middle of your mat.

2. Hug your knees tightly into your chest, squeezing your body as closely as possible. Make yourself as small as you can be. (See illustration 27.)

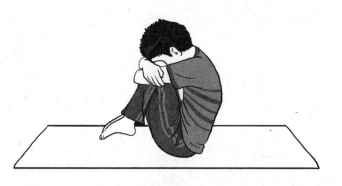

Illustration 27: From sitting to reclining—smallest you

3. Slowly open your body, stretching your arms and legs as far away as you can, making yourself as big as you can be, and lower down until you are lying flat on your back. (See illustration 28.)

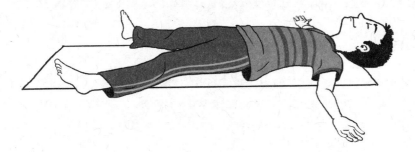

Illustration 28: From sitting to reclining—biggest you

4. Now try repeating this a few times. From your back, pull up to sit and curl into a small ball. Then lower down again. The more times you do this, the stronger your core will get, and the more relaxing your reclining activity will feel.

Bringing Energy Up (Gently): Waking Up Your Body

This simple activity asks your child to bring his attention to each part of his body and move it through its full range of motion, starting with his feet and moving up to his head. You can do this quickly or slowly based on your child's attention span and interest level.

1. Start in mountain pose (see chapter 6), and bring your attention to your toes. Explore how they move. Wiggle them, pick them up, spread them out, and then place them back down.

2. Now explore the rest of your feet and ankles. Roll them in circles, point and flex your feet, and make any other possible movements.

3. Move up your legs and find your knees. Pick them all the way up one at a time, and then bend them as deeply as you can. What other movements are your knees responsible for? Consider jumping, lunging, squatting.

4. Keep moving up your body to your hips and explore how they move. Make big circles with your legs, open and close your hips, maybe give each leg a good shake.

5. Continue moving up your body, pausing at each joint to move it any way that feels good. Be playful and creative as you figure out how many ways your body has to move.

Bringing Energy Down: Rag Doll Pose

This is a basic forward fold that provides an easy way to rest and let your energy settle down.

1. Begin in mountain pose (see chapter 6).

2. Slowly fold forward, letting your body be soft.

3. Let your arms hang down and your head be heavy. (See illustration 29.)

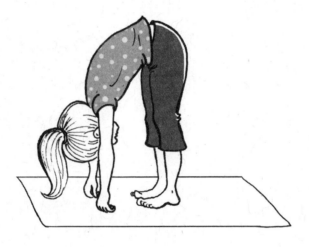

Illustration 29: Rag doll pose

4. If your hamstrings feel tight, you can bend your knees a little bit.

5. Try swaying gently from side to side and forward and back.

6. Take a few full breaths, and then as you breathe in, roll very slowly back up to standing.

Coming Back to Neutral: Simple Twist

This simple, gentle twist can be practiced between any of the activities. It provides a grounding, neutralizing energy that can aid in your transitions.

1. Begin seated with your legs crossed, or straight out in front of you. Sit up tall.

2. Lift your arms up to the sky, getting as tall as possible while keeping your shoulders relaxed.

3. Bring your right hand to your left knee and your left fingertips to the floor behind you.

4. Sit up tall as you inhale, and then exhale and gently pull your knee with your right hand and twist to the left, looking out over your left shoulder.

5. Keep the right side of your seat firmly on the ground and your shoulders soft. (See illustration 30.)

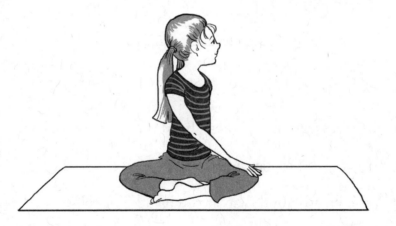

Illustration 30: Simple twist

6. Switch sides when you are ready.

Getting Creative

You know your child best, and once you get used to these practices, feel free to swap out activities in any sequence for ones that you think would work better for your child, or try creating your own sequences together. Just keep in mind the bell curve structure, and consider starting with a calm activity, bringing the energy up, and then slowly bringing the energy back down so that the ending of your session is quiet and relaxing.

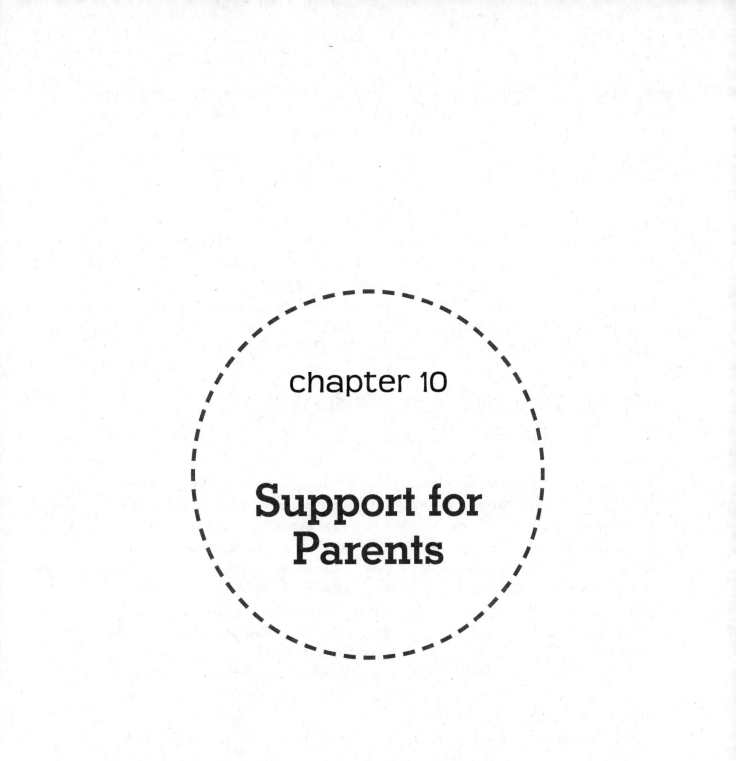

chapter 10

Support for Parents

Parenthood is a beautiful, challenging, exciting, frustrating, mind-boggling journey. So is childhood! As you and your child work together, compassion is the most important place to return to when things get hard: compassion for yourself, and compassion for your child. A yoga practice of your own can be a tremendous tool in this work of parenting, and it will be an anchor in surprising and inspiring ways.

The following contribution was written by a LFY student named Kate Gilbane. Kate is a parent of three children, one of whom struggles with ADHD and dyslexia. Her exact experience is unique, but the impact of her practice on her parenting is a recurring truth that I have heard many times from parents of children with and without specific challenges. Her contribution here of ten guidelines for compassionate parenting is a gift for any parent, and each idea incorporated into your life and the life of your family will bring you greater peace and improved relationships.

Practice Yoga, Parent Better

"Chandler... Chandler!... CHANDLER!!" I ask Chandler to climb down off the back of the couch, which she uses as a balance beam. I ask her where she left her shoes (for the umpteenth time) and she stares blankly back at me. I watch her get out of the car and completely forget to close the door behind her. I walk into her bedroom and see clothes strewn all over the floor, clothes that haven't even been worn. I ask her over and over again to put on her coat and backpack so we can leave for school. I watch her agonize over a simple homework assignment or a handwritten thank-you note. I see how incessantly she moves her body—squirming, jerking, bouncing, tapping her foot—in an effort to concentrate on reading or fine-motor skills. I observe as she gets up from the table four or five times during a meal, unable to remain seated. I watch her hopeful insistence turn to fury upon being told she may not do exactly what she wants to do (like having a lemonade stand or launching an online jewelry-making business) right this very instant. I try desperately to remain calm while she melts down in a maelstrom of emotions ("big, messy feelings"), collapsing on the floor, kicking and screaming, or even trying to hit me.

I went to my first yoga class about twelve years ago. I felt something I'd never felt before: A sense of balance, lightness, and ease in my body. I felt peaceful, calm, and yet highly aware. It's the first time that I can actually remember listening and responding to my body. By showing up for class, I was allowing myself to receive the benefits of yoga's healing powers. I went back to class as often as I could. Now yoga inspires everything I do every single day—especially the way I parent.

Parenting can be an incredible balance between utter frustration/despair and profound joy/gratitude. Yoga has taught me how to ride that emotional roller coaster without falling off. Yoga is always there for me with the same basic tools I need to stay grounded. It has made the "downs" of the parenting ride much more manageable and the highs, because I am fully present for them, more thrilling. In yoga, they say, "Do your practice and the rest will follow." I say, "Do your practice and better parenting will follow."

Chaos has always been my biggest trigger. Growing up as the oldest of five children, I was highly sensitive to the constant chaos around me and felt a need to control and "perfect" things in order to save my family. Over time and practice, yoga has taught me to let go. Letting go is still a conscious effort for me, rather than something that comes naturally or easily. The more I practice yoga, the more relaxed I feel. The less I practice, the more I tend to slip into anxious, neurotic behavior. Jenn Harper once clarified in a Little Flower Yoga training that the goal of the teacher is not to control the class but to loosen her grip enough to allow each child to have his or her own experience.

The same principle obviously applies in parenting. The more I can loosen my grip as a mom, the more space I can hold for my three children to emerge as individuals, to experience the life they are here to experience, to be who they are. I see myself getting in their way when grasping for perfection and order. I see what a hindrance that assertion of control is to their mental, emotional, and spiritual development. I see the beauty that unfolds when I become more of a loving witness. Yoga helps me allow it.

My husband and I call our lowest moments "breakdowns for breakthroughs" and, honestly, I don't think you can have the latter without the former. When I'm really struggling as a parent, I remind myself that I must contract sometimes in order to then expand. When I get angry, I remind myself that anger is an impetus for change. If I find myself angry about something, I need to look very closely and figure out what type of change would turn that situation around. When I am challenged in any way as a parent or otherwise, a yoga class *always* helps me diffuse the emotional charge and re-find my way by providing comfort, reassurance, and connection to my true self, where there are always ideas, resources, and better perspectives.

Greater self-awareness around my own parenting is one of the benefits of my yoga practice. Because of yoga, I am decidedly self-reflective. I pay more attention to what I do, what I say, how I say it, and so on. Yoga helps clear the clutter from my head so I can witness my own behavior with clarity and be honest with myself about when, where, and how I want to make changes/improvements. Yoga has taught me to ask questions like, "What *does* my parenting look like? What kind of parent am I striving to become?" Yoga shows me how tremendous progress can be made by taking baby steps—on the mat or in my daily life—as I move closer to my goals. Maybe it's a more enthusiastic and physically affectionate way of greeting my daughter in the morning (despite being up all night with her newborn baby brother) or maybe it's the way I take ever deeper breaths when I'm upside down in wheel pose—both practices help open my heart and bring me a little closer to *samadhi* (bliss).

Yoga philosophy inspires my most meaningful parenting ideals—to be honest (with my children), to be generous (with my children), to be loving and kind and never violent (toward my children), to be devoted to a higher power (all of us). And the more I talk to my kids about this stuff, the more available they are for it. It's so natural for them and yet we need to offer them the opportunity to see it in action, ask questions about it, take ownership of what resonates for them. I know my kids want desperately to be heard, and when I come back from yoga class I am always a better listener. I can also draw on that feeling by simply setting the intention and using my breath to center myself and become available. I am certain that the more I actually listen to my kids, the more love they feel from me.

Patience, flexibility, finding a sense of calm no matter what is happening around me (or if that doesn't work, then leaving the room for a few minutes!), the ability to turn struggle into meditation or an intense breathing exercise, the ability to reconnect with the flow of my own life (like the flow of a class) rather than resisting it, focusing on gratitude rather than the negative—these are the types of life skills that have transformed and empowered my parenting. The surrender changes everything—in a difficult pose on my mat or in the kitchen at 5 p.m. when my kids are hungry, exhausted, and pushing all my buttons. When I can step back and see what's really happening when things get messy, call it something ("meltdown hour"), and *not* take it personally, I can continue to move through it and accomplish what needs to be accomplished (without losing my temper.) From 5 to 6 p.m. may not be my favorite time of day, but when I take the presumptuous dread and judgment out of it, I may be surprised. Who knows? If nothing else, it feels really good to handle this time without resistance, the way I intended to handle it—to be calm, cool, and collected. I can't do it every time, but thanks to my yoga practice, my track record's getting a lot better. This *is* my yoga practice.

Last spring, my oldest child was diagnosed with mild ADHD and mild dyslexia. As I began to acknowledge all the implications of that, I relied even more heavily on my yoga practice to remind me that this was all going to work out just fine. Today, I cannot imagine myself as a parent or a kids' yoga teacher (in training) without this invaluable experience. What better way for me to become more skillful at engaging with and appreciating a child who struggles with self-regulation and focus than to parent one? My daughter has taught me to let go in ways that I never imagined possible and to see the beauty in something that our society still insists on deeming unruly and inappropriate. It's not always easy for me to hold space for my daughter, but yoga always helps me step back and see that she's teaching me exactly what I need to know to be a really good parent/teacher. As I find myself saying to Chandler things like, "While it may be frustrating to feel like your body is restless and out of control sometimes, you'd *never* want to trade that incredible amount of energy that runs through you. Think about all the amazing things you can do with that energy. It's enviable!" I am able to convince myself and her, at the same time, that it is truly a gift.

A Guide to Compassionate Parenting

One of my favorite quotes from a training with Jenn is: "Life will teach our kids that life isn't fair. We need to show them that when life's not fair, we're on their side." With this in mind, here are some guidelines for compassionate parenting that have helped me navigate this challenging journey.

1. **Meet your own basic needs for healthy food, water, sleep, and exercise.** Sleep is huge. If I am tired, my whole day is a struggle—which is okay once in a while but not on a regular basis. Think of it as one of your primary responsibilities to your children to get the amount of rest you need to be patient and energetic.

2. **Talk to your kids about your own self-care/spiritual practice** (yoga, massage, workouts, reading, educational classes, etc.). Show them how you carve out time for it and how much it enhances your life when you do.

3. **Get yourself and your kids outdoors.** As difficult as it is to get three young children dressed in winter gear and out the door, that fresh air and change of scene (which hopefully incorporates nature) seems to be one of the most reliable mood enhancers.

4. **When you need a break, give *yourself* a time-out.** Removing yourself from the emotionally charged environment can often help you re-center and get back on track. Take a few deep breaths, reinstate your parenting intention, and come back to the situation with a fresh sense of purpose.

5. **When your children are angry or otherwise upset, encourage them to practice a physical/emotional release**, like stomping or punching out their angry feelings. Give them permission to cry and let their big, messy emotions come spilling out. Let them go to their rooms and use loud, abrasive, inflammatory language, as long as no one can hear them. Let them scribble on a big piece of paper or blackboard to "show" how angry they are. Or hold up a big sofa cushion so they can hit it. I have my daughter lie down on the floor in the playroom when she's furious and put her legs up in the air. I throw a bean bag chair toward her and she catches it with her feet and pushes it back toward me with all her might. This really works to diffuse anger for both of us.

6. **Do what you say you're going to do.** Be as reliable and consistent as possible, and when you aren't, then acknowledge it. Your kids need to be able to trust you to be real with them, to tell the truth, and to admit it when you mess up. Try to ensure that nannies, babysitters, and other caregivers do the same.

7. **Focus on the positive and encourage your kids to do the same** (not when they're upset, however). Have a simple gratitude/self-reflection practice. My kids love to "talk about their day" at bedtime. It's such a nice way to review what happened, the highlights, the teachable moments, the important people, and to set goals, and so on. We keep a whiteboard in the kitchen to record all the acts of kindness/helpfulness that happen at home. It's the "Good Stuff" list and the kids love it!

8. **Try not to rush your kids.** Being in a hurry creates so many problems. Mindfulness goes right out the window. On the flip side, when you have

time to spare because you're early or you've scheduled in "unscheduled time" to just be, kids are so happy and relaxed. It's like when you make the effort to really listen—amazing things can happen.

9. **Acknowledge that, much of the time, kids don't know how to act.** Be compassionate about that and make thoughtful decisions about how to respond. Maybe they need to be left alone, or maybe they need some guidance. Make sure you don't call attention to negative behavior, unless it's necessary. When kids are embarrassed or uncomfortable, they may act uncharacteristically, but don't make it worse for them by shaming them. It's highly counterproductive.

10. **When you have important things to discuss with your kids, carve out an appropriate time and place to do so.** Give them the benefit of being well rested and in a good mood so that they can respond optimally. Think about how you would feel in their shoes. Who wants to discuss anything when they're frustrated or otherwise emotionally charged? Wait until your kids feel good and their ability to reason and empathize will be there.

—Kate Gilbane

Your Personal Practice

If it is at all possible, get yourself to a yoga class of your own, even if it's only once in a while. In addition, do everything you can to create small moments for yourself to take full breaths, notice how you are feeling, and make mindful decisions. All of the activities in this book will support your own well-being, not just your child's.

There are many different styles of yoga, and not all of them are a good fit for every person. When you are looking for a class for yourself, make sure to stay open-minded, and if one class or one teacher doesn't feel like a good fit, try another until you find one that makes you feel supported, accepted, challenged, relaxed, and happy. During class, follow the guidelines that you follow with your child: Don't feel pressured to do anything that doesn't feel right, take breaks when you need them, remember that *you* are more important than the yoga, and take care of yourself without embarrassment or shame. Ask questions when you need to, and stick around for *savasana*.

Compassionate Behavior Management

When your child is struggling with emotional regulation and poor attention skills, it's almost a certainty that your home life will be filled with challenging behavior that is up to you to manage. Dealing with frustrating behavior, setting boundaries, and helping your child develop his capacity for inner discipline is not necessarily a talent that blossomed in you at his birth. Dealing compassionately and effectively with difficult behavior is a skill that you can learn, practice, and improve.

The single most relevant truth that I have embraced when dealing with negative behavior (in both children and adults) is to remember that, for the most part, when people feel good, they act good, and when people feel bad (particularly when they feel bad about themselves), their behavior reliably gets worse. When your child makes you angry, frustrated, or terrified, and you are about to speak to them, ask yourself if what you are about to say is going to make them feel better or worse. If what's about to come out of your mouth is going to make your child feel worse, you can be pretty sure that their behavior isn't going to improve anytime soon. Take a minute, take a breath, and think of something, anything, you can say to help your child feel better in that moment. What might make him feel better? Knowing that you are on his side! If your child knows that you are on his side, no matter what happens, then he knows that he is safe. He knows that he is loved, and whatever needs to come next (a conversation, a consequence, a negotiation, a confession) becomes a little less scary, a little more comprehensible, and a lot more effective. You might even try waking up each morning and thinking to yourself, *What can I do or say in the next hour or two that will make my child feel good about himself?* See if that preemptive action helps set you up for a better day.

Of course, no matter how hard you work at making your child feel good, there will be daily challenges to address. There are lots of resources out there that offer strategies and suggestions, many of them listed in the Recommended Reading section that follows, but the three books that I recommend you take a look at first are:

The Whole-Brain Child: 12 Revolutionary Strategies to Nurture Your Child's Developing Mind by Daniel J. Siegel and Tina Payne Bryson

How to Talk So Kids Will Listen and Listen So Kids Will Talk by Adele Faber and Elaine Mazlish

Everyday Blessings: The Inner Work of Mindful Parenting by Myla Kabat-Zinn and Jon Kabat-Zinn

Don't Forget!

As you read this book, the books recommended above, and whatever other advice you seek out, remember that every child is unique, and the relationship between you and your child is one that nobody else can fully understand. If suggestions go against your instincts and something doesn't feel right, really roll it around in your mind before you decide if you will give it a try. Make sure that your actions are authentically motivated, and be confident in your ability to love fully. Shake off any pressure, doubt, and fear keeping you from fully enjoying the short time that your child will be a kid. Trust yourself. Your child needs you. You need your child.

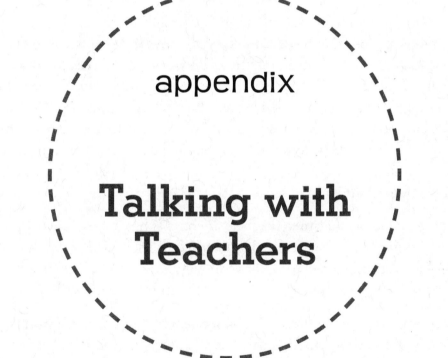

appendix

Talking with
Teachers

When your child is struggling, particularly if those struggles are manifesting as behavior problems, it's easy to develop an adversarial relationship with her teachers. Here are some suggestions:

- **Communicate:** Be in touch with your child's teacher when things are going well, not just when there are difficulties. Say thank you, share stories, be friendly. Fill him or her in on what's happening with your child without embarrassment. A teacher can only support your kid if he or she knows what is going on.

- **Cultivate a partnership:** If something is working at home, let your child's teacher know. Most will be happy to integrate your tools into the classroom, but (and this is an important but) make sure that when you talk with a teacher you do so in a considerate way. Assume that the teacher has expertise that is valuable. Don't suggest that you know best—remember that this person is a professional and a human being capable of feeling threatened and defensive. Rather, say that you know your child best, and that you need the teacher's help to meet your child's needs. A great way to show the teacher that you respect him or her is to ask for his or her suggestions and whether there is anything that he or she is working on in the classroom that you can support in your home. Focus on creating a consistent and predictable environment for your child.

- **Introduce one idea at a time:** Teachers are busy. They are usually overworked and trying to do many things at once. If you come to them with a whole big program for your kid, they might feel too overwhelmed (and maybe a little insulted) to integrate any of it. Be clear, specific, and simple with your requests.

- **Try not to internalize your child's challenges:** Blaming yourself won't help. Don't be embarrassed to show emotion in front of a teacher, and try to recognize that by acknowledging your child's challenges the teacher is not blaming you or judging you. Emotional conversations can easily make both parties defensive—try to recognize the difference between defensiveness and advocating for your child.

- **Involve the school counselor:** School counselors have so much to offer—advice, resources, mediation, and support. Take advantage of this and include them in your conversations with your child's teacher early on in your relationship. If you are struggling in your relationship with a teacher, the counselor can be a great source of advice.

- **Involve your child:** It can be very powerful to include your child in the conversations with her teacher. This empowering step allows your child to feel invested in the plan of action. It also allows you an opportunity to facilitate greater understanding between your child and the teacher.

Recommended Reading

There are many wonderful resources available to help you discover your strengths as a parent, learn more about your child, and live a rich and rewarding family life. Included in the following list are some of my favorites. While it's tempting to go right for the parenting books, I recommend you spend a little time developing your own personal practice with books such as *Mindfulness for Beginners,* by Jon Kabat-Zinn, and *Relax and Renew,* by Judith Lasater. For more resources and up-to-date additions to this recommended reading list, visit our blog: http://littlefloweryoga.com/blog.

Building Emotional Intelligence: Techniques to Cultivate Inner Strength in Children by Linda Lantieri. Boulder, CO: Sounds True, 2008.

Eastern Body, Western Mind: Psychology and the Chakra System as a Path to the Self by Anodea Judith. Berkeley, CA: Celestial Arts, 2004.

Emotional Intelligence: Why It Can Matter More Than IQ by Daniel Goleman. New York: Bantam Books, 2006.

Everyday Blessings: The Inner Work of Mindful Parenting by Myla Kabat-Zinn and Jon Kabat-Zinn. New York: Hyperion, 1997.

Hold On to Your Kids: Why Parents Need to Matter More Than Peers by Gordon Neufeld and Gabor Maté. New York: Ballantine Books, 2005.

How to Talk So Kids Will Listen and Listen So Kids Will Talk by Adele Faber and Elaine Mazlish. New York: Avon Books, 1999.

Mindfulness for Beginners: Reclaiming the Present Moment—and Your Life by Jon Kabat-Zinn. Boulder, CO: Sounds True, 2012.

Parenting from the Inside Out: How a Deeper Self-Understanding Can Help You Raise Children Who Thrive by Daniel J. Siegel and Mary Hartzell. New York: J.P. Tarcher/Penguin, 2003.

Planting Seeds: Practicing Mindfulness with Children by Thich Nhat Hanh. Berkeley, CA: Parallax Press, 2011.

Raising an Emotionally Intelligent Child: The Heart of Parenting by John Gottman and Joan DeClaire, with foreword by Daniel Goleman. New York: Simon & Schuster, 1998.

Relax and Renew: Restful Yoga for Stressful Times by Judith Lasater. Berkeley, CA: Rodmell Press, 1995.

Recommended Reading

Scattered Minds: A New Look at the Origins and Healing of Attention Deficit Disorder by Gabor Maté. Toronto: Vintage Canada, 1999.

Still Quiet Place: Mindfulness for Young Children (audio CD) by Amy Saltzman. CD Baby, 2007.

The Healing Path of Yoga: Time-Honored Wisdom and Scientifically Proven Methods That Alleviate Stress, Open Your Heart, and Enrich Your Life by Nischala Joy Devi. New York: Three Rivers Press, 2000.

The Heart of Yoga: Developing a Personal Practice by T. K. V. Desikachar. Rochester, VT: Inner Traditions International, 1999.

The Mindful Child: How to Help Your Kid Manage Stress and Become Happier, Kinder, and More Compassionate by Susan Kaiser Greenland. New York: Free Press, 2010.

The Mindfulness Prescription for Adult ADHD: An 8-Step Program for Strengthening Attention, Managing Emotions, and Achieving Your Goals by Lidia Zylowska, foreword by Daniel J. Siegel. Boston: Trumpeter, 2012.

The Relaxation and Stress-Reduction Workbook for Kids: Help for Children to Cope with Stress, Anxiety and Transitions by Lawrence Shapiro and Robin Sprague, foreword by Matthew McKay. Oakland, CA: New Harbinger, 2009.

The Secret Power of Yoga: A Woman's Guide to the Heart and Spirit of the Yoga Sutras by Nischala Joy Devi. New York: Three Rivers Press, 2007.

The Whole-Brain Child: 12 Revolutionary Strategies to Nurture Your Child's Developing Mind by Daniel J. Siegel and Tina Payne Bryson. New York: Delacorte Press, 2011.

Yoga Calm for Children: Educating Heart, Mind, and Body by Lynea Gillen and Jim Gillen. Portland, OR: Three Pebble Press, 2007.

Yoga for Children: 200+ Yoga Poses, Breathing Exercises, and Meditations for Healthier, Happier, More Resilient Children by Lisa Flynn. Avon, MA: Adams Media 2013.

Yoga Nidra: The Meditative Heart of Yoga by Richard Miller. Boulder, CO: Sounds True, 2005.

30 Essential Yoga Poses: For Beginning Students and Their Teachers by Judith Lasater. Berkeley, CA: Rodmell Press, 2003.

References

Arch, J., and M. Craske. 2006. "Mechanisms of Mindfulness: Emotion Regulation Following a Focused Breathing Induction." *Behavior Research and Therapy* 44(12): 1849–1858.

Aton, S., J. Seibt, and M. Frank. 2009. "Sleep and Memory." *eLS*. doi:10.1002/97804700 15902.a0021395.

Berger, D., E. Silver, and R. Stein. 2009. "Effects of Yoga on Inner-City Children's Well-Being: A Pilot Study." *Alternative Therapies in Health and Medicine* 15(5): 36–42.

Devi, N. J. 2007. *The Secret Power of Yoga: A Woman's Guide to the Heart and Spirit of the Yoga Sutras.* New York: Three Rivers Press.

Diamond, A. and K. Lee. 2011. "Interventions Shown to Aid Executive Function Development in Children 4 to 12 Years Old." *Science* 333(6045): 959–964.

Diekelmann, S., and J. Born. 2010. "The Memory Function of Sleep." *Nature Reviews Neuroscience* 11, 114–126. doi:10.1038/nrn2762.

Flook, L., S. Smalley, M. Kitil, B. GAlla, S. Kaiser-Greenland, J. Locke, E. Ishijima, and C. Kasari. 2010. "Effects of Mindful Awareness Practices on Executive Functions in Elementary School Children." *Journal of Applied School Psychology* 26 (1): 70–95.

Froeliger, B., E. Garland, and F. McClernon. 2012. "Yoga Meditation Practitioners Exhibit Greater Gray Matter Volume and Fewer Reported Cognitive Failures: Results of a Preliminary Voxel-Based Morphometric Analysis." *Evidenced-Based Complementary and Alternative Medicine.* doi: 10.1155/2012/821307.

Goldin, P., and J. Gross. 2010. "Effects of Mindfulness-Based Stress Reduction on Emotion Regulation in Social Anxiety Disorder." *Emotion* 10(1): 83–91.

Goldin, P., W. Ramel, and J. Gross. 2009. "Mindfulness Meditation Training and Self-Referential Processing in Social Anxiety Disorder: Behavioral and Neural Effects." *Journal of Cognitive Psychotherapy* 23(3): 242–257.

Goleman, D. 1995. *Emotional Intelligence: Why It Can Matter More Than IQ*. New York: Random House Publishing Group.

James, W. 1950. *Principles of Psychology*. New York: Dover Publications.

Jensen, P., and D. Kenny. 2004. "The Effects of Yoga on the Attention and Behavior of Boys with Attention-Deficit/Hyperactivity Disorder (ADHD)." *Journal of Attention Disorders* 7(4): 205–216.

Kabat-Zinn, Jon. 1994. *Wherever You Go, There You Are: Mindfulness Meditation in Everyday Life*. New York: Hyperion.

Luders, E., A. Toga, N. Lepore, and C. Gaser. 2009. "The Underlying Anatomical Correlates of Long-Term Meditation: Larger Hippocampal and Frontal Volumes of Gray Matter." *Neuroimage* 45(3): 672–678.

Luders, E., F. Kurth, E. Mayer, A. Toga, K. Narr, and C. Gaser. 2012. "The Unique Brain Anatomy of Meditation Practitioners: Alterations in Cortical Gyrification." *Frontiers in Human Neuroscience* 6:344.

Maté, G. 2000. *Scattered: How Attention Deficit Disorder Originates and What You Can Do About It*. New York: Plume.

McGonigal, K. 2012. "Your Brain on Meditation." *Mindful Magazine*, www.mindful.org /the-science/neuroscience/your-brain-on-meditation.

Mendelson, T., M. Greenberg, J. Dariotis, L. Gould, B. Rhoades, and P. Leaf. 2010. "Feasibility and Preliminary Outcomes of a School-Based Mindfulness Intervention for Urban Youth." *Journal of Abnormal Child Psychology* 38(7): 985–994.

Muris, P., C. Meesters, H. Merckelbach, A. Sermon, and S. Zwakhalen. 1998. "Worry in Normal Children." *Journal of the American Academy of Child & Adolescent Psychiatry* 37(7): 703–710.

Napoli, M., P. Krech, and L. Holley. 2005. "Mindfulness Training for Elementary School Students: The Attention Academy." *Journal of Applied School Psychology* 21 (1): 99–125.

National Sleep Foundation. "Children and Sleep." Accessed April 2013. www.sleepfounda tion.org/article/sleep-topics/children-and-sleep.

References

Oberle, E., K. Schonert-Reichl, M. Lawlor, and K. Thomson. 2012. "Mindfulness and Inhibitory Control in Early Adolescence." *The Journal of Early Adolescence* 32(4): 565–588.

Roeser, R., and S. Peck. 2009. "An Education in Awareness: Self, Motivation and Self-Regulated Learning in Contemplative Perspective." *Educational Psychologist* 44(2): 119–136.

Sadeh, A., R. Gruber, and A. Raviv. 2003. "The Effects of Sleep Restriction and Extension on School-Age Children: What a Difference an Hour Makes." *Child Development* 74(2): 444–455.

————. 2002. "Sleep, Neurobehavioral Functioning, and Behavior Problems in School-Age Children." *Child Development* 73(2): 405–417.

Semple, R., J. Lee, D. Rosa, and L. Miller. 2010. "A Randomized Trial of Mindfulness-Based Cognitive Therapy for Children: Promoting Mindful Attention to Enhance Social-Emotional Resiliency in Children." *Journal of Child & Family Studies* 19(2): 218–229.

Siegel, D., and T. Bryson. 2011. *The Whole-Brain Child: 12 Revolutionary Strategies to Nurture Your Child's Developing Mind.* New York: Delacorte Press.

Silverman, W., A. La Greca, and S. Wasserstein. 1995. "What Do Children Worry About? Worries and Their Relation to Anxiety." *Child Development* 66(3): 671–686.

Slagter, H., R. Davidson, and A. Lutz. 2011. "Mental Training as a Tool in the Neuroscientific Study of Brain and Cognitive Plasticity." *Frontiers in Human Neuroscience* 5(17).

Wahlstrom, K. 2010. "School Start Time and Sleepy Teens." *Archives of Pediatrics & Adolescent Medicine* 164 (7): 676–677.

Woolery, A., H. Myers, B. Sternlieb, and L. Zeltzer. 2004. "A Yoga Intervention for Young Adults with Elevated Symptoms of Depression." *Alternative Therapies in Health and Medicine,* 10(2): 60–63.

Jennifer Cohen Harper, MA, E-RCYT, is a leading voice in the children's yoga community. She is the founder and director of New York-based Little Flower Yoga and The School Yoga Project, cofounder and board vice president of the Yoga Service Council, and an active member of the International Association of Yoga Therapists. Harper leads the well-respected Little Flower Yoga Teacher Training for Children program, provides therapeutic yoga classes to children and families, and frequently collaborates with other organizations to bring yoga for children to places as diverse as tent cities in Port au Prince, Haiti, and FAO Schwarz retail stores in New York City.

Foreword writer **Daniel J. Siegel, MD,** is an internationally acclaimed author, award-winning educator, and child psychiatrist. He is currently a clinical professor of psychiatry at the UCLA School of Medicine where he also serves as a co-investigator at the Center for Culture, Brain, and Development and co-director of the Mindful Awareness Research Center. He is also the executive director of the Mindsight Institute, an educational center devoted to promoting insight, compassion, and empathy in individuals, families, institutions, and communities. His books include *Mindsight, The Developing Mind, The Mindful Brain, The Mindful Therapist, Parenting from the Inside Out,* and *The Whole-Brain Child.* He lives in Los Angeles, CA, with his wife and two children.